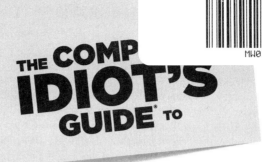

Using Your Computer—For Seniors

by Paul McFedries

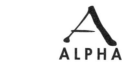

A member of Penguin Group (USA) Inc.

ALPHA BOOKS

Published by the Penguin Group

Penguin Group (USA) Inc., 375 Hudson Street, New York, New York 10014, USA • Penguin Group (Canada), 90 Eglinton Avenue East, Suite 700, Toronto, Ontario M4P 2Y3, Canada (a division of Pearson Penguin Canada Inc.) • Penguin Books Ltd., 80 Strand, London WC2R 0RL, England • Penguin Ireland, 25 St. Stephen's Green, Dublin 2, Ireland (a division of Penguin Books Ltd.) • Penguin Group (Australia), 250 Camberwell Road, Camberwell, Victoria 3124, Australia (a division of Pearson Australia Group Pty. Ltd.) • Penguin Books India Pvt. Ltd., 11 Community Centre, Panchsheel Park, New Delhi—110 017, India • Penguin Group (NZ), 67 Apollo Drive, Rosedale, North Shore, Auckland 1311, New Zealand (a division of Pearson New Zealand Ltd.) • Penguin Books (South Africa) (Pty.) Ltd., 24 Sturdee Avenue, Rosebank, Johannesburg 2196, South Africa • Penguin Books Ltd., Registered Offices: 80 Strand, London WC2R 0RL, England

Copyright © 2012 by Paul McFedries

All rights reserved. No part of this book may be reproduced, scanned, or distributed in any printed or electronic form without permission. Please do not participate in or encourage piracy of copyrighted materials in violation of the author's rights. Purchase only authorized editions. No patent liability is assumed with respect to the use of the information contained herein. Although every precaution has been taken in the preparation of this book, the publisher and author assume no responsibility for errors or omissions. Neither is any liability assumed for damages resulting from the use of information contained herein. For information, address Alpha Books, 800 East 96th Street, Indianapolis, IN 46240.

THE COMPLETE IDIOT'S GUIDE TO and Design are registered trademarks of Penguin Group (USA) Inc.

International Standard Book Number: 978-1-61564-161-1
Library of Congress Catalog Card Number: 2011936772

14 13   8 7 6

Interpretation of the printing code: The rightmost number of the first series of numbers is the year of the book's printing; the rightmost number of the second series of numbers is the number of the book's printing. For example, a printing code of 12-1 shows that the first printing occurred in 2012.

Printed in the United States of America

Note: This publication contains the opinions and ideas of its author. It is intended to provide helpful and informative material on the subject matter covered. It is sold with the understanding that the author and publisher are not engaged in rendering professional services in the book. If the reader requires personal assistance or advice, a competent professional should be consulted.

The author and publisher specifically disclaim any responsibility for any liability, loss, or risk, personal or otherwise, which is incurred as a consequence, directly or indirectly, of the use and application of any of the contents of this book.

Most Alpha books are available at special quantity discounts for bulk purchases for sales promotions, premiums, fund-raising, or educational use. Special books, or book excerpts, can also be created to fit specific needs.

For details, write: Special Markets, Alpha Books, 375 Hudson Street, New York, NY 10014.

Publisher: *Marie Butler-Knight*
Editorial Director: *Mike Sanders*
Executive Managing Editor: *Billy Fields*
Senior Acquisitions Editor: *Tom Stevens*
Development Editor: *Lynn Northrup*
Senior Production Editor: *Janette Lynn*
Copy Editor: *Lisanne V. Jensen*
Cover Designer: *William Thomas*
Book Designers: *William Thomas, Rebecca Batchelor*
Indexer: *Angie Martin*
Layout: *Ayanna Lacey*
Senior Proofreader: *Laura Caddell*

ALWAYS LEARNING   PEARSON

For my parents

Contents

Part 1: Getting Comfy with Your Computer 1

1 A Few Computer Basics 3
   Getting to Know Your Computer 4
      The Case, Monitor, Keyboard, and Mouse 4
      A Closer Look at the Case 5
      A Quick Peek Under the Hood 9
   Setting Up Your Computer 11
      Organize Your Work Area 11
      Connect the Components 12
   Starting Your Computer 20
   Connecting Even More Devices 21
      CD or DVD Disc 21
      Memory Card 23
      Flash Drive 24
      Digital Camera or Camcorder 24
      Media Player 25
      External Hard Drive 25

2 Getting to Know Windows 27
   What Is Windows? 27
   A Tour of the Screen 29
      The Desktop 30
      The Taskbar 30
   A Few Mouse and Keyboard Fundamentals 31
      Basic Mouse Maneuvers 31
      Common Keyboard Conveniences 34
   Shutting Down and Restarting Your Computer 36
      Putting Your Computer to Sleep 36
      Restarting Your Computer 38

3 Installing and Running Programs 39
   Installing a Program 40
      Installing Windows Live Essentials Programs 40
      Installing a New Program 42

	Uninstalling a Program 44
	Uninstalling a Windows Live Essentials Program 44
	Giving a Program the Heave-Ho 45
	Launching a Program 46
	A Look at the Start Menu 47
	Navigating the Start Menu 50
	Working with Programs 53
	Pull-Down Menus 53
	Toolbars 57
	Special Cases: WordPad, Paint, and Windows Live 59
	Dialog Boxes 60
	Switching from One Program to Another 62
	Quitting a Program 64

4 Dealing with Documents 67

What Is a Document? 68
Creating a New Document 68
Entering and Editing Document Text 69
Saving Your Work 73
  Saving a New Document 74
  Saving an Existing Document 75
  Organizing Your Documents 76
  Creating a Folder 77
  Creating a Copy of a Document 78
Closing a Document 79
Opening an Existing Document 79
Locating Documents on Your Computer 80

5 Playing with Photos, Music, and Movies 83

Getting Photos onto Your Computer 84
  Transfer Photos from a Digital Camera 84
  Scan a Photo 88
  Transfer Photos from a Memory Card 90
Photo File Formats 92
Viewing Photos 94
  Looking Through Your Photos 95
  Watching a Photo Slide Show 98

Contents   vii

	Fixing Your Photos 99
	Straighten a Photo.. *100*
	Remove Red Eye *101*
	Crop Out Unwanted Elements *103*
	Copying Photos to a CD or DVD 104
	Working with Other Types of Media 106
	Listening to an Audio CD *106*
	Copying Music from an Audio CD *107*
	Watching DVD Movies.. *109*
6	**Troubleshooting Your Computer** **113**
	Backing Up Your Computer...114
	Backup to an External Hard Drive *115*
	Configuring the Backup..*116*
	Creating a System Repair Disc *118*
	How to Troubleshoot a Problem..119
	Determine the Source of the Problem *119*
	Try Some General Troubleshooting Tips................................ *121*
	Run Windows's Troubleshooters *122*
	Getting Troubleshooting Help 124
	Online Resources.. *124*
	The Remote Control Route... *125*
	Recovering from a Problem 128
	Recovering a Lost File *128*
	Recovering from Program Crashes *130*
	Recovering Using System Restore... *133*
	Recovering Your System from a Backup.................................*135*

Part 2: Making Your Computer Easier to Use **139**

7   **Circumventing Visual Challenges** **141**

      Making Things Bigger 142
         Adjust the Screen Resolution.. *142*
         Scale the Screen... *144*
         Zoom In on the Screen... *147*
      Making Things Easier to See 148
         Switch to a High-Contrast Screen *149*
         Make the Mouse Pointer Easier to See...................................*151*
         Make Dialog Boxes Easier to See... *152*

　　　　　Removing Distractions 153
　　　　　Hearing What's on the Screen.................................. 154

8　Surmounting Hearing Challenges 157
　　　　Speakers or Headphones? 158
　　　　Adjusting the Volume 159
　　　　　Adjust the Overall System Volume............................ 160
　　　　　Adjust an Application's Volume................................ 161
　　　　　Balance Your Headphones 163
　　　　　Equalize the Volume... 164
　　　　Getting Visual Cues to Screen Activity 165
　　　　　Turn On Visual Notifications for Sounds.................. 166
　　　　　Display Text Captions for Spoken Dialog 167

9　Overcoming Physical Challenges 169
　　　　Making the Mouse Easier to Use................................ 170
　　　　　Control the Mouse Pointer with Your Keyboard....... 170
　　　　　The Need for Speed: Making Mouse Keys Faster 173
　　　　　Easier Mouse Dragging... 174
　　　　　Easier Window Selection 176
　　　　　Prevent Automatic Window Arranging..................... 177
　　　　Making the Keyboard Easier to Use 179
　　　　　Press Multiple-Key Commands One Key at a Time ... 180
　　　　　Sticky Situations: Sharing Your Computer 181
　　　　　Avoid Unwanted Keystrokes..................................... 183
　　　　　Ignore Multiple Keystrokes 184
　　　　　Control Multiple Keystrokes..................................... 185
　　　　Keeping Notifications Onscreen Longer.................... 186
　　　　Controlling Your Computer with Voice Commands.......... 188

Part 3: Using Your Computer to Go Online 193

10　Setting Up a Network and Internet Access 195
　　　　Researching Internet Service Providers 196
　　　　　Do It with Dial-Up... 198
　　　　　Head Down the Broadband Highway........................ 200
　　　　Connecting the Equipment... 201
　　　　　Dial-Up Details... 201
　　　　　Broadband Basics... 202

Setting Up the Connection 204
    Create the Connection *205*
    Future Connections *209*
Severing the Connection 211
Going Wireless 211
    Setting Up the Wireless Connection *212*
    Configuring the Wireless Router *214*
    Making the Wireless Connection *217*

11   Surfing the Web 219
Taking a Look at Internet Explorer 220
Web Page Navigation Basics 224
    Saving Your Favorite Sites *226*
    Surfing with Tabs *228*
    Downloading Files to Your Computer *229*
Searching for Information on the Web 230
Some Tasks You Can Do on the Web 231
    Share Photos *232*
    View Maps and Get Directions *234*
    Read the News *235*
    Research Your Family History *238*
    Find Recipes and Cooking Tips *239*
    Locate Health Information *240*

12   Exchanging Email 243
Getting Started with Windows Live Mail 244
Setting Up Your Internet Email Account 244
    The High Road: Quick Account Setup *244*
    The Low Road: Configuring an Account By Hand *245*
Touring Windows Live Mail 247
Sending an Email Message 249
    Compose and Send a Message *249*
    Use the Contacts List *251*
    Email a Photo *252*
    Email Other Types of Files *253*
Getting and Reading Email Messages 254
    Get Your Messages *255*
    Read Your Messages *255*

Handle File Attachments.. *257*
Do Something with a Read Message....................................... *257*
Creating Folders to Store Your Messages............................... 259

13   Getting the Most from Online Shopping 261
Online Shopping: The Pros and Cons 262
Doing Your Research.. 263
Products.. *263*
Prices.. *266*
Online Retailers.. *268*
Buying Things Online 270
Booking a Trip... 271
Using Online Coupons.. 274

14   Connecting with Family and Friends................................ 279
Understanding Social Networking 279
Finding the Right Social Network................................... 281
Setting Up and Using a Facebook Account........................... 283
Creating a Facebook Account...................................... *284*
Configuring Your Facebook Profile................................ *286*
Making Friends... *287*
Handling a Friend Request *292*
Update Your Status on Facebook *293*
Share Photos on Facebook... *295*
Share Links on Facebook.. *295*

Part 4: Staying Safe Online 297

15   Playing It Safe on the Web 299
Avoiding Viruses... 300
Keeping Spyware at Bay.. 303
Heeding Windows's Warnings 306
Secure Surfing: Some General Tips 307
Even More Ways to Protect Yourself on the Web................... 310
Creating Secure Passwords *310*
Should You Give Out Your Credit Card Information? *312*
Deleting Your Browsing History................................... *313*
Browse Privately *316*
Block Pop-Up Windows.. *317*

16	**Keeping Your Email Safe and Sound**	**321**
	Protecting Yourself Against Email Viruses	322
	Some General Ways to Avoid Email Viruses	*322*
	Windows Live Mail's Antivirus Settings	*323*
	Shielding Yourself from the Scourge of Spam	325
	Junk ... Spam ... What's Up with These Messages?	*325*
	How to Avoid Spam	*327*
	Using the Junk Mail Filter to Can Spam	*329*
	Setting the Junk Email Protection Level	*329*
	Identifying Hoaxes and Other Annoyances	332
	Identifying Good Guys and Bad Guys	334
	Specifying Safe Senders	*334*
	Blocking Senders	*335*
17	**Avoiding Scams**	**337**
	Understanding Phishing Scams	338
	Phishing Email Messages	*339*
	Windows Live Mail's Anti-Phishing Tools	*341*
	Phishing Websites	*342*
	Internet Explorer's Anti-Phishing Tools	*343*
	Preventing Identity Theft	345
	Protecting Yourself from "419" Scams	347
	Preventing Fraud When Shopping Online	349
	General Considerations	*349*
	The Best Way to Pay	*350*
	Avoiding Online Auction Fraud	*352*
	Check Overpayment Scams	*354*
	Bogus Health Products	*354*
	"Free" Offers That Aren't So Free	*355*

Appendixes

A	Glossary	359
B	Online Resources for Seniors	373
	Index	377

Introduction

For those of us who have been on the earth for a while, it isn't hard to recall a time when it was unusual for a household to have its own computer. Heck, those of us who are of a certain age grew up during a time when it was simply inconceivable that anyone would want (or could even afford) a computer in the home. Back in 1943, IBM head honcho Thomas Watson famously said, "I think there is a world market for maybe five computers."

Now, of course, you'd be hard-pressed to find a household that does *not* own a computer. That's because it took everyone about five minutes to realize that computers make a lot of sense, particularly for young people and working families who have young kids. But what about seniors? Does it make sense for older adults to own a computer? Well, the numbers speak for themselves. According to the United States Bureau of Labor Statistics, between 2000 and 2008, the percentage of people age 65 to 74 who owned a computer more than doubled from 31 to 64 percent—and for folks age 75 and older, computer ownership more than *tripled* during that time, from 13 to 42 percent.

In other words, seniors are flocking to computers like so many swallows to Capistrano. Why? Because they've realized that computers have a lot to offer in making their lives easier, more interesting, and more fun. Whether it's writing a letter to the editor of the local newspaper, viewing photos of your grandkids, or making your own greeting cards, a computer makes many tasks simpler and faster. And if you go online, your computer becomes your gateway to the vast riches and social connections that are available through the World Wide Web, email, and more.

However, using a computer isn't all beer and skittles. They can be difficult to set up, confusing to use, and intimidating for the uninitiated. And, of course, things such as the screen, the mouse, and the keyboard present special challenges to aging eyes, ears, and hands.

If these negative aspects of using a computer are holding you back, then you've come to the right place. Welcome to *The Complete Idiot's Guide to Using Your Computer—For Seniors*. In this book, you learn everything you need to know (but thankfully, not *everything* there is to know) about using a computer: from understanding the various bits and pieces that make up the machine, to getting the hang of Windows, and to setting up your computer to work around any physical challenges you may face. And we'll even have a bit of fun while we're at it.

How This Book Is Organized

The Complete Idiot's Guide to Using Your Computer—For Seniors is organized into four reasonably sensible parts. To help you locate what you need fast, here's a summary of what you'll find in each part:

Part 1, Getting Comfy with Your Computer, gets you off to a gentle start by giving you the skinny on what a computer is and what Windows is and giving you easy-to-follow instructions for basic tasks such as installing programs, working with documents and photos, and solving problems.

Part 2, Making Your Computer Easier to Use, can help you overcome issues with eyesight, hearing, and physical dexterity. You learn how to make it easier to see things on the screen, how to better hear the sounds that emanate from your computer, and how to make the mouse and keyboard less of a challenge to use.

Part 3, Using Your Computer to Go Online, devotes five chapters to the internet. You'll learn step by step how to get connected to the internet, how to surf the World Wide Web with Internet Explorer, how to use internet email, how to shop online, and how to use social networking to stay in touch with family and friends.

Part 4, Staying Safe Online, closes the book with three chapters that will help you avoid problems while you're using the internet. You learn how to keep viruses and other web tribulations at bay, minimize junk messages and other email miscreants, and protect yourself from various online scams.

I round out your PC education by offering two helpful appendixes: a glossary of technical terms and a list of senior-friendly websites for you to check out.

Help Along the Way

I've liberally sprinkled the book with features that will make it easier for you to understand what's going on. Here's a rundown:

- Menus, commands, and dialog box controls that you have to select, keys you have to press, and stuff that you type will appear in a **bold font**.

- When I tell you to select a menu command, I separate the various menu and command names with commas. For example, instead of saying, "Click the **Format** menu, then click **Theme**, and then click **Colors**," I just say this: "Click **Format, Theme, Colors**."

- Many Windows commands come with handy keyboard shortcuts, and most of them involve holding down one key while you press another key. For example, in some applications you save your work by holding down the **Ctrl** key, pressing the **S** key, and then releasing **Ctrl**. I'm *way* too lazy to write all that out each time, so I just add a plus sign (+) between the two keys, like so: **Ctrl+S**.

I've also populated each chapter with different kinds of sidebars that give you tips, cautions, definitions, and other tidbits of information:

Good to Know!

These sidebars show you useful tweaks that enable you to supercharge your system and take control over various aspects of your machine.

What Can Go Wrong?

These sidebars warn you about possible PC pitfalls and tell you how to avoid them.

Definition

These sidebars give you definitions of new words suitable for use at cocktail parties and other social gatherings, where a well-timed bon mot can make you a crowd favorite.

By the Way

These sidebars give you extra information about the topic at hand, provide you with techniques for making things work easier, and generally make you a more well-rounded computer user.

Acknowledgments

Many thanks to everyone who worked with me on this book, including Senior Acquisitions Editor Tom Stevens, Development Editor Lynn Northrup, Senior Production Editor Janette Lynn, Copy Editor Lisanne Jensen, and Technical Editor Mark Hall.

Special Thanks to the Technical Reviewer

The Complete Idiot's Guide to Using Your Computer—For Seniors was reviewed by an expert who double-checked the accuracy of what you'll learn here, to help us ensure that this book gives you everything you need to know about using your computer. Special thanks are extended to Mark Hall.

Mark Hall has been editing technical books for 21 years, with over 250 edited and 2 co-authored titles to his credit. For more than 25 years Mark has been the technical services manager for the Community Colleges of Spokane. He and his wife Brenda have four children.

Trademarks

All terms mentioned in this book that are known to be or are suspected of being trademarks or service marks have been appropriately capitalized. Alpha Books and Penguin Group (USA) Inc. cannot attest to the accuracy of this information. Use of a term in this book should not be regarded as affecting the validity of any trademark or service mark.

Getting Comfy with Your Computer

Part 1

My overall goal in this book is to help you get productive with your computer. And by "getting productive," I mean not only getting things done but also getting online, getting creative, and generally getting the most from your new electronic roommate. Now, I'll let you in on a not-so-little secret: the key to getting productive with your computer in general, and with Windows in particular, is becoming comfortable with a few basic operations and features. Once you're familiar with these fundamentals, everything else you do with your computer will be significantly easier.

So getting comfy with the nuts and bolts of your computer and Windows is what happens in Part 1. You learn about the computer's sundry parts, how to set up your computer and work area, basic tasks such as using the mouse and keyboard, how to work with programs and windows, how to create and save documents, how to work with photos and music, and much more.

A Few Computer Basics

Chapter 1

In This Chapter

- Learning about the main parts of your computer
- Setting up your computer and work area
- Getting your computer up and running
- Connecting devices to your computer

My goal in this book is to show you not only how to use your computer but also how to make your computer do things that are useful (and occasionally just plain fun). Over the years that I've used computers myself and taught other people how to use them, one of the main things I've learned is that before you can learn *how* to use a computer, it helps immensely if you know *what* you're working with.

Fortunately, that doesn't mean you need to know all the details of what's happening inside the computer. Techies care about all that, but you certainly don't have to. In that sense, using a computer is a bit like driving a car: you don't have to know the inner workings to make it do something worthwhile. To that end, I'll just focus on the main things you can see—with a few tidbits about some of the things you can't see, which will prove useful down the road (you'll have to trust me on this).

Getting to Know Your Computer

Let's start this tour of computer basics by looking at what computer geeks like to call *hardware:* the physical components that make up your system. This includes the computer itself as well as everything that gets attached to it.

The Case, Monitor, Keyboard, and Mouse

Beginning at the beginning, Figure 1.1 shows a typical computer setup and points out the relevant parts.

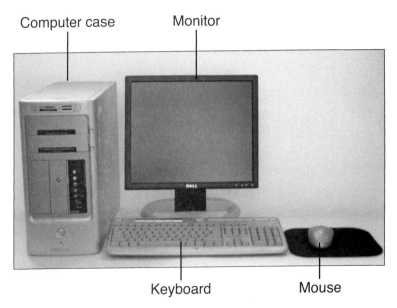

Figure 1.1: A typical computer setup and its components.

Here's a summary of what you see:

- **Computer case**   The inside of this big box is the home of all the electronic doohickeys and doodads that enable the computer to do its thing (and which, happily, you'll almost certainly never have to see or work with directly). So what's inside the case is really the computer per se, which is why you'll often hear people calling it the *system unit*. The outside of the case is populated with various switches and slots, and I'll tell you a bit about all that in the next section.

- **Monitor**   This TV-like part is what the computer uses to display its text, images, and other data. Some folks also call it the *video display*, and the rectangular part that shows the data is called the *screen*.

- **Keyboard**   This typewriter-like part is what you use to enter information (such as a letter or a list). In some cases, you also use the keyboard to type instructions for the computer to follow. You learn how to use the keyboard in Chapter 2.

- **Mouse**   This odd part works as a kind of hand-operated pointing device that you use to select things on the screen that you want to work with, as well as to move things here and there on the screen. I'll show you how the mouse works in Chapter 2.

A Closer Look at the Case

The irony of using a computer is that the most important part—that is, the computer case—is the part you'll work with the least. While you're working with your computer, you'll be staring at the monitor, typing away on the keyboard, and using the mouse.

However, that doesn't mean you should ignore the case. It really is, as I've said, the main part of the computer—so it pays to take a few seconds and get to know the case a bit more intimately. To that end, Figure 1.2 shows the front of a typical computer case and points out the most important features.

> **By the Way**
>
> Figure 1.2 shows a typical case, but it's by no means the most common layout. Computer manufacturers seem to almost throw the various parts around randomly, so although your case will have all or most of the features I show in Figure 1.2, it's a fairly sure bet that they'll appear in different places.

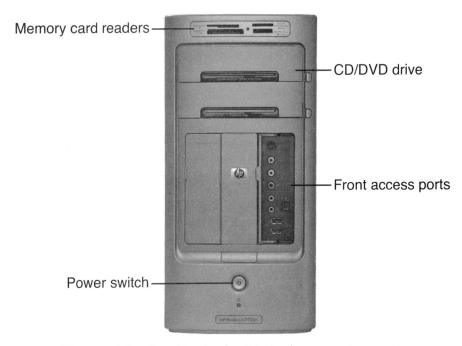

Figure 1.2: The front of a typical computer case.

Let's take a look at what we're seeing here:

- **Memory card readers** You use these slots to insert *memory cards*, a type of portable storage device that typically works with digital cameras. See Chapter 5 to learn more about memory cards.
- **CD/DVD drive** You use this slot to insert CDs or DVDs, which look similar to music CDs. Again, see Chapter 5 for more details.

Chapter 1: A Few Computer Basics

- **Front access ports**   These are extra ports that are similar to those on the back of the computer (discussed next) but are easier to reach.

- **Power switch**   When your computer is turned off, you press this button to turn on the power.

The front of the case only has a few widgets to furrow your brow, but the back of the case is an entirely different gizmo ballgame. As you can see in Figure 1.3, the back is positively festooned with an odd variety of holes and plugs.

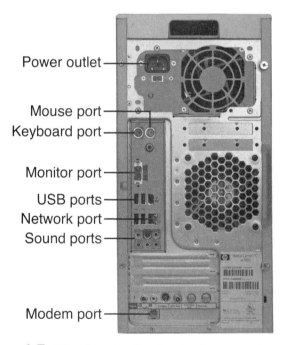

Figure 1.3: The back of a typical computer case.

Let's knock some sense into these knickknacks:

- **Power outlet**   This is where the computer's power cord plugs in.
- **Keyboard port**   This is where you plug in the keyboard, although many a modern keyboard plugs into a USB port instead.
- **Mouse port**   This is where you plug in the mouse, although again, the typical modern mouse plugs into a USB port instead.
- **Monitor port**   This is where you connect your monitor.
- **USB ports**   You use these ports to plug in devices that use the *Universal Serial Bus* (USB) connector. Keyboards, mice, printers, digital cameras, and many other devices use USB connectors.
- **Network port**   This is where you connect your computer to a wired network or an internet modem, as described in Chapter 10.
- **Sound ports**   You use these ports to connect sound devices to your computer. If you have external speakers, they connect to the Line Out (green) port; if you have a microphone, you connect it to the Mic In (pink) port.
- **Modem port**   If you're going to connect to the internet using a dial-up modem, this is the port you'll use to connect the phone cord.

I know this is a lot to digest at this early stage, but here are three reasons not to worry too much about any of this back-of-the-case stuff right now:

- As you saw in Figure 1.2, the front of most computer cases comes with a few front-access ports—particularly USB and sound ports—so you may never have to use any of the back ports.
- You'll learn a lot more about making these physical connections later in this chapter, so if the details are a bit fuzzy right now, things should clear up considerably in just a bit.

- Although there are perhaps a couple dozen ports shown in Figure 1.3, the vast majority of computer setups use only a fraction of these: the power outlet, the monitor port, a USB port or two, and the speaker port.

A Quick Peek Under the Hood

As I mentioned earlier, you don't need to be a mechanic to drive a car—and you don't need to be an electrical engineer to use a computer. Three cheers for that! However, when you think about it, you *do* need to know a tiny bit about how an engine works to operate a car successfully. For example, it helps to know that an internal combustion engine uses gas, so you'll be sure to fill up the tank every now and then!

Your computer won't run out of gas, of course, but there are a few internal things you should know about to get the most from your computer and to better understand what's happening as you work with the machine. Fortunately, there are just three main internal dinguses that you should be on familiar terms with:

- **Central processing unit** This part—also known as the *CPU*, *microprocessor*, or simply the *processor*—runs the show inside your computer. The CPU's main job is to coordinate the flow of data throughout the computer (which is why some folks describe the CPU as its "brain"). So—with a few exceptions—no matter what happens on your computer, the CPU has a hand in it somehow. Press a key on your keyboard, for example, and the signal goes through the keyboard port to the processor, which then passes along the signal to the rest of the system. The CPU also keeps itself busy by performing math and logic calculations, sending data to and from memory and the hard drive, processing hardware and software instructions, and lots more.

- **Hard drive** This device—feel free to also call it a *hard disk*—is your computer's main storage area. When you first got your computer, it already had Windows installed on the hard drive, and any other programs you install (see Chapter 3) will also get stored on the hard drive. Also, anything you create on your computer—letters, email messages, or greeting cards—gets stored on the hard drive.

- **Memory** Your computer's memory—also called *RAM*, which is short for *random access memory*—is a temporary work area that the CPU uses to hold data when you run a program. Memory is much faster than the hard drive, so when the CPU needs data, it grabs the data from the hard drive and then loads it into memory. Why not just load the entire hard drive into memory? Because, for technical reasons, all computers have a maximum amount of memory they can use—usually about 4GB, or gigabytes—while most hard drives hold at least a hundred times that amount of data.

By the Way

Hard drive (and memory) capacities are measured in *gigabytes* (GB). To understand this, first know that a single character—the letter *A*, the number *7*, or the asterisk symbol (*)—is represented inside the computer by a single *byte* of data. A thousand bytes is called a *kilobyte;* a thousand kilobytes is called a *megabyte;* and a thousand megabytes is a gigabyte.

As a helpful analogy, think of your computer as a carpenter's workshop divided into two areas: a storage space (the hard drive) for tools and materials and a work area (the memory) where the carpenter (the CPU) actually uses these things. The problem is that your computer's "workspace" is much smaller than its "storage space." For a carpenter, a small workspace limits the number of tools and the amount of wood that can be used at any one time. For a CPU, it limits the number of programs and data files it can load.

Fortunately, all this happens out of sight and without the slightest intervention on your part, so you don't have to worry about a thing as you use your computer.

Setting Up Your Computer

Did you get yourself a new computer, or have you inherited a "pre-owned" computer from a friend or family member? Is that computer just lying around in pieces, waiting for someone to put everything together? If so, then you've come to the right place—because in this section, I show you how to set up your work area and then connect all the components.

Organize Your Work Area

Before getting to the nuts and bolts of the actual computer setup, let's take a few minutes to consider the setup of your work area. After all, using a computer is a much more pleasant experience if you're comfortable and if you set things up so that sitting, typing, using the mouse, and even just looking at the screen won't cause physical problems.

First, where should everything go? Bearing in mind that you may have only a limited number of places to put your computer, the location you choose should be clean, dry, and temperate (not too hot and not too cold; computers don't like temperature extremes). The area should also be well lit, preferably from above or behind the monitor to prevent glare. And, of course, you'll need one or more electrical outlets nearby.

Next, make sure that the desk you're using to hold your computer is sturdy and stable. It should also have a large enough surface to hold all the computer's desktop components (such as the monitor, keyboard, and mouse), as well as any books, papers, and other materials you may use as you work.

You also need to give some thought to the chair you'll use. If you pick a chair that's uncomfortable or poorly designed, it can affect your work performance. You need a chair that has a contoured seat and good lower-back support. It should also have mechanisms to adjust the seat height as well as the angle of both the seat and the back support.

For maximum comfort and safety, you can apply the principles of *ergonomics* to your work area and work habits:

- Adjust the chair height so that your forearms are parallel to the floor when you type and your eyes are level with the top of your monitor.
- Sit up straight in your chair with your feet flat on the floor.
- When you're in the middle of a long session with the computer, at least once every hour you should get out of your chair and stretch or go for a walk.
- You can buy many accessories that ensure good ergonomics. For example, to help keep your wrists straight, you can use wrist rests below your keyboard and mouse. An adjustable keyboard tray helps ensure that your keyboard is at the proper height. You can use a monitor stand to ensure that the monitor height is correct. Finally, to keep your feet flat, you can use a footrest.

Definition

Ergonomics is a set of principles and practices for setting up a computer work area to help to maximize comfort and safety.

Connect the Components

A typical computer comes with a fair number of parts, which can be intimidating—but putting everything together isn't as hard as it looks, as you will see in this section.

If your computer is brand new, first remove each component and double-check the packing list to ensure that you received everything you ordered. If the computer arrived on a cold day, give the components a couple hours to warm up to room temperature. At this stage, don't plug anything into an electrical outlet.

Your next order of business is deciding where to put the computer case, and that depends on which style of case you have:

- **Tower** This style of case is tall with a relatively narrow base (see Figure 1.2 earlier in the chapter). In this case (pun semi-intended), it's best to place the computer on the floor, either under or beside the desk. Your monitor, keyboard, and mouse sit on the desk. (I should mention at this point that you'll soon be connecting devices to the ports in the front and back of the case, so don't squirrel the case too far under the desk for now or you won't be able to reach the ports without contorting yourself in ways not intended by nature.)

- **Desktop** This style of case is short with a relatively wide base. As the name implies, this type of case goes on the desk and you place the monitor on top of it (and the keyboard and mouse in front of it).

You're now ready to assemble your system by connecting the devices to the appropriate ports on the back of the computer case (or the front, if your case has front-access ports).

Good to Know!

On most computers, the ports on the back of the case are color-coded to match the device plugs. Also, most device plugs fit into only one type of port, so it isn't possible to plug a device into the wrong port.

Connect the Monitor

Let's start with the monitor, which comes with two cables: a power cord and a video cable. You can leave the power cord unplugged for now. The video cable is a bit less straightforward because there are two main types of connectors.

One connection type is called *VGA*, and it has a D-shaped plug (see Figure 1.4) that you can insert into the port with the same shape (see Figure 1.5) on the back of the computer.

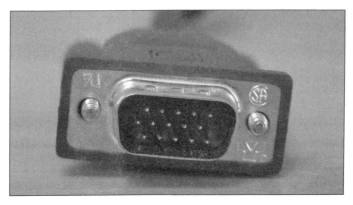

Figure 1.4: Your monitor may come with a video cable that uses this type of connector.

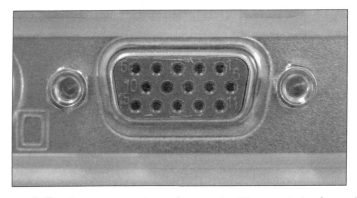

Figure 1.5: The connector shown in Figure 1.4 plugs into this type of port on the back of the computer.

The other main connection type is *DVI*, and it uses a long, narrow plug similar to the one shown in Figure 1.6. It plugs into the corresponding port on the back of the computer, which will look similar to the one shown in Figure 1.7.

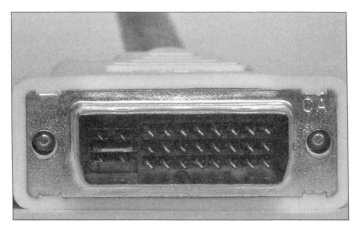

Figure 1.6: Many modern monitors use a video cable with this type of connector.

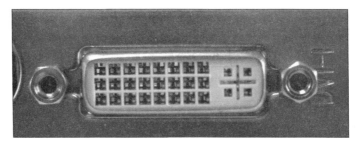

Figure 1.7: The plug in Figure 1.6 connects to this type of port on the back of the computer.

Connect the Keyboard and Mouse

When it comes to connecting your keyboard and mouse, there are three possibilities:

- Most keyboards and mice made in the last few years connect to the computer via USB. If that's what you have (or if you're not sure), see "Connect Your USB Devices" later in this chapter.

- *Wireless* keyboards and mice are quite common these days. If yours don't have any cords dangling from them, then you have wireless models. In this case, you only need to connect the part that communicates with the keyboard and mouse—a device called a *transceiver*—to a USB port (so again, see "Connect Your USB Devices").

- Older keyboards and mice use the special connectors shown in Figure 1.8. You can't tell in black-and-white, but the one on the left is the mouse connector, and it's green—while the one on the right is the keyboard connector, and it's purple. These connect to the corresponding green and purple ports on the back of the computer (see Figure 1.9).

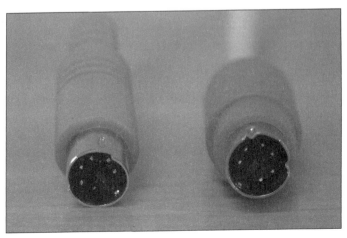

Figure 1.8: Some old-style mouse (left) and keyboard (right) connectors.

Chapter 1: A Few Computer Basics   **17**

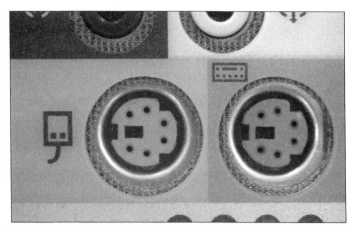

Figure 1.9: The connectors in Figure 1.8 plug into the ports of the same color on the back of the computer.

What Can Go Wrong?

The old-timey mouse and keyboard connectors can be a bit tricky to insert. See the rectangular holes inside the ports in Figure 1.9? Each connector has a plastic tab of the same size and shape, so in each case you need to carefully align the tab with the hole in the port.

Connect the Printer

This one's easy because all printers of recent vintage connect via a USB cable, so see "Connect Your USB Devices" for the details. Leave the printer's power cord unplugged for now.

Connect the Sound System

If your computer comes with a set of speakers, one of them will have a green RCA-style jack, as shown in Figure 1.10. This connects to the corresponding round, green port (sometimes labeled Line Out) on the back (or sometimes the front) of the computer, shown in Figure 1.11 (it's the port on the right). The second speaker will also have an RCA jack, and this connects to a port on the back of the first speaker. Finally, if you have a microphone, it will most likely have a pink RCA jack that connects to the corresponding pink port (sometimes labeled Mic In or just Mic) on the back of the PC (it's the port on the left in Figure 1.11).

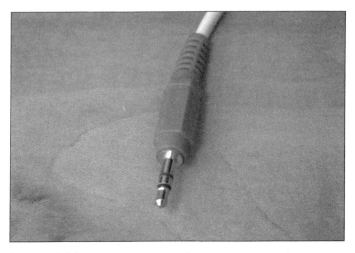

Figure 1.10: Your PC speakers come with a green RCA-style jack.

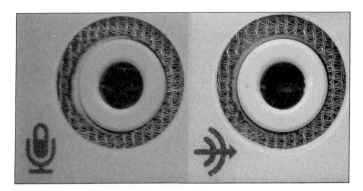

Figure 1.11: The speaker jack in Figure 1.10 connects to the green Line Out port on the back of the computer.

Connect Your USB Devices

As I mentioned earlier, all recent computers ship with anywhere from four to eight USB ports, and many have an extra two to four on the front panel. This means you can connect lots of USB devices—which is a good thing because so many devices now come with USB connectors, including the following:

- Keyboard
- Mouse
- Printer and/or document scanner
- Digital camera or camcorder
- Media player (such as an iPod)
- External hard drive

Figure 1.12 shows a USB connector, and Figure 1.13 shows a collection of USB ports.

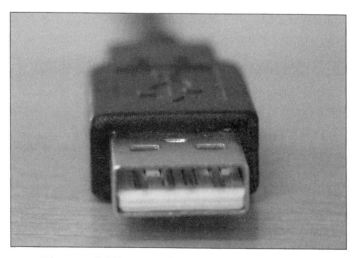

Figure 1.12: Your basic USB connector.

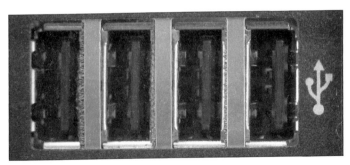

Figure 1.13: Most computers come with a bunch of USB ports. Note the road-sign-for-aliens symbol on the right, which helps you identify USB ports and plugs.

As you can see in Figure 1.12, each USB connector has a strip of plastic inside, as does each USB port (see Figure 1.13). The only way to successfully insert a USB connector into a USB port is to line up these plastic strips so that they're opposite each other.

Plug In the Power Cords

With all your devices connected, you can now plug in the power cords for all your devices. Ideally, you should use a surge protector or power strip that has a built-in surge protector. This ensures that a lightning strike won't damage the sensitive innards of your computer.

Starting Your Computer

Now that you've connected your devices to your computer and everything's plugged in that needs to be plugged in, you're ready to start your computer for the first time. First, turn on all your computer's peripheral devices, including the monitor, the printer, and the speakers (if you have any). Now, press your computer's power button, or flip its on/off switch.

What Can Go Wrong?

If nothing happens when you turn on your system, check the computer's power cord connections at both ends to ensure that you have properly plugged in the cord. Also, check that the surge protector or power strip is plugged in and turned on. Finally, ensure that you have turned on your monitor.

If you're starting up a brand-new computer, each manufacturer has its own setup program that runs the first time. This usually takes just a few minutes, and you're typically asked for information such as your name, the username that you want to use when you log on to Windows (your first name is a good choice here), a password, and a name for your computer. If you're not sure how to go about creating a strong and secure password, I give you some pointers in Chapter 15.

After the setup program ends, Windows appears and you're ready to roll. Note that each time you start your computer in the future, you'll need to enter your password—so be sure to remember the password you chose when you set up Windows.

Connecting Even More Devices

You'll start learning about Windows in Chapter 2. For now, I'd like to take just a bit more of your time to go through a few other bits of hardware that you may come across during your computing journey.

CD or DVD Disc

Your computer probably comes with a CD or DVD drive to insert a CD or DVD and access the files on the disc. To insert a disc in the drive, first press the button on the front of the drive. (This button varies rather alarmingly from drive to drive, so it's tough for me to be any more specific.) This causes the disc tray to slide out. Now, remove the disc from its case or sleeve (be sure to touch only the edges of the disc) and then place the disc, writing-side up, in the drive's disc tray (see Figure 1.14). Now, close the disc tray—usually either by pressing the drive button again or by giving the tray a gentle push.

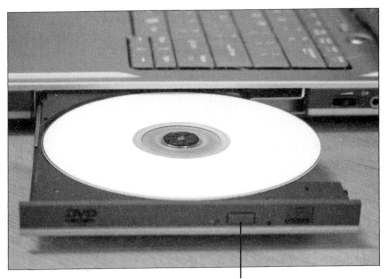

Figure 1.14: Open the drive's disc tray and place the disc onto the tray.

 Good to Know!

Oddly, some CD and DVD drives don't have disc trays at all. Instead, you see a narrow slot in the front of the drive. Insert your disc into that slot until it catches and inserts itself the rest of the way. When you're done, press the drive button to eject the disc.

Memory Card

If your computer comes with a built-in memory card reader (or if you connected a card reader to the PC via USB), then you can use it to access the contents of memory cards. Unfortunately, most card readers come with four or more slots, so how in the name of Pete is a person supposed to know which one to use? It's not straightforward, unfortunately, but there are a couple ways to get your bearings:

- On most card readers, each slot is accompanied by text that tells you which kinds of memory cards will fit. So if you see MMC (or MultiMedia Card) on the card itself, look for the slot that includes "MMC" in the label.

- The slots are different shapes and sizes, which sounds like a bad thing (more confusing!), but it's not because any memory card will only fit correctly into a single slot. So if you're really not sure which one to use, try inserting the card (writing-side up) until you get a good fit.

Figure 1.15 shows a CompactFlash memory card inserted into a reader.

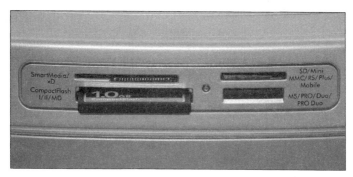

Figure 1.15: A memory card inserted into a slot in a memory card reader.

Flash Drive

A *flash drive* (also called a *thumb drive*) is a device for storing files. They're convenient because although they're small (about the size of a few sticks of gum), they can hold a decent amount of data. As a bonus, you don't need extra equipment such as a card reader because all flash drives connect via your old friend, the USB port. Remove the cap to expose the USB connector (see Figure 1.16), then plug the drive straight into the nearest available USB port.

> **By the Way**
>
> Some flash drives don't use a cap. Instead, you expose the USB connector by sliding a tab on the side of the drive.

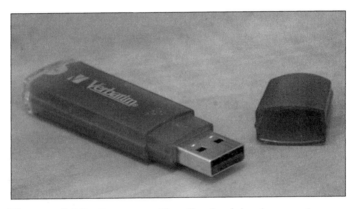

Figure 1.16: Remove the flash drive's cap to see the USB connector.

Digital Camera or Camcorder

If you have a digital camera or a digital camcorder, you'll want to connect it to your computer to access your photos and videos. I talk about this in detail in Chapter 5, but for now you should know how to connect a digital camera. Fortunately, this is much easier than it used to be; for a few years now, cameras and camcorders have been using USB to connect.

First, dig out the USB cable that came with your camera and take a good look at it. You'll notice that one end uses a standard-issue USB connector while the other end uses something completely different. It's this latter end that plugs into the camera, so look for a port on the camera that looks like it has the right shape and size to accept the cable. (Some cameras hide the port under a rubber or plastic flap.) Plug the other into a USB port on your computer, then turn on the camera.

Media Player

A *media player* is a device such as an iPod or iPad that plays music, movies, videos, and other entertaining pastimes. To load up your media player with media, you need to connect it to your computer. Most media players (perhaps even all of them) support USB, so use the cable that came with the device to insert one end into the player and the other into a free USB port.

External Hard Drive

Earlier, you learned about the hard drive that resides inside your computer and serves as a home for all your digital stuff. But just as a home may also require an external building, such as a garage or shed to store even more stuff, your computer may also need external storage. You've seen several external storage devices so far, including memory cards, flash drives, and CD/DVD drives—but they all have relatively limited storage space. For some major external-storage real estate, you need to look at an external hard drive.

Why bother, you ask? The best reason is for making all-important backups of your documents. The ideal place to store these backups is some kind of external storage area, because if your computer goes down for the count, at least all your previous files are stored safely on the external storage device. An external hard drive is the ideal choice here because you can easily get one that's large enough to contain a backup of your entire system (see Chapter 6 for backup details).

Most external hard drives are—you guessed it—USB devices, so you can plug the hard drive into any available USB port (if you have any left, that is!).

The Least You Need to Know

- The computer case is the most important part of the system because inside it contains the CPU, the hard drive, and the memory—and outside, it contains the slots and ports you use to connect devices.
- The CPU is perhaps the most important component because it controls and monitors everything that happens within your computer.
- For the best experience with your computer, choose a sturdy desk, a comfortable chair with good support, and a location that's well lit and temperate.
- Practice good ergonomics by adjusting the chair height so that your forearms are parallel to the floor when you type and your eyes are level with the top of your monitor.
- When setting up your computer, leave everything unplugged from a power source while you make the connections.
- Many devices make connections easy by supporting USB, including keyboards, mice, printers, document scanners, digital cameras and camcorders, media players, and external hard drives.

Getting to Know Windows

Chapter 2

In This Chapter

- Understanding this thing called Windows
- Touring the Windows screen
- Getting a grip on the mouse
- Solving the mysteries of the keyboard
- Shutting down or restarting your computer safely

After all that hardware talk in Chapter 1, things take a softer turn here in Chapter 2. With your computer now up and running and the Windows screen beckoning you, it's time to knock some sense into this Windows business. To that end, this chapter introduces you to Windows and takes you on a tour of the screen. If you've never used Windows before, you'll appreciate the mouse and keyboarding lessons that come next. I'll close by showing you how to shut down Windows for the night as well as restart your computer.

What Is Windows?

Now, you might be asking yourself (or, more to the point, you might be asking *me*), "How can I figure out Windows if I don't even know what it is?" That's an excellent question! Windows is what computer know-it-alls call an *operating system*, a fancy way of saying that Windows controls the overall operation of your computer. I said something similar about the CPU in Chapter 1, so let me explain a bit more.

The CPU controls almost every aspect of the hardware side of your computer, so in that sense it's like the chief engineer who runs the engine room on a ship. Windows is more like the crew who takes care of every other aspect of the ship's operation, from the captain to the helmsman to the stewards. In practical terms, this means that Windows handles things such as displaying what you see on the screen, ensuring that whatever you type on your keyboard gets sent to the correct program, and making sense of anything you do with the mouse.

Perhaps Windows' most important job is to manage the programs on your system. When you want to start a program, you tell Windows which one you want, and it performs all the necessary behind-the-scenes tasks needed to get the program running. Windows also ensures that the program has enough memory, fetches data from (and sends data back to) the hard drive as needed by the program, and takes care of shutting down the program when you tell Windows you're done with it.

Windows also acts as a go-between for you and your devices. For example, when you connect a new device to your computer, Windows makes sure that the device gets set up correctly. Similarly, if you ask a device to do something—say, you ask your printer to print a document—it's Windows that does the actual asking (or really, *telling*).

It's important to remember that the vast majority of this goes on sight unseen, so you never have to worry about most of it. All you have to do is learn enough about Windows to make it do the things you want it to do, and you'll certainly do that in this book.

A Tour of the Screen

The screen shown in Figure 2.1 is typical of the face that Windows 7 presents to the world. If you're new to Windows 7, you need to get comfortable with the lay of the Windows land. To that end, let's examine the territory you now see before you, which I divide into two sections: the desktop and the taskbar.

> **By the Way**
>
> Your screen may have a different look than the one shown in Figure 2.1, depending on how your computer manufacturer chose to set up your machine or if you're using an earlier version of Windows, such as Vista or XP.

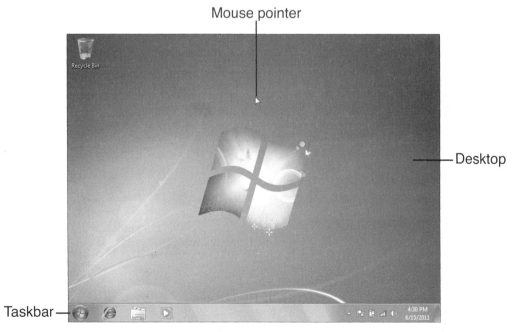

Figure 2.1: The Windows 7 landscape.

The Desktop

Ivory-tower computer types enjoy inventing metaphors for the way the rest of us use a computer. The idea is that more people will put up with a computer's shenanigans if using the computer reflects the way we do things in real life.

For Windows, the metaphor of choice is the humble *desktop*. That is, you're supposed to think of the Windows screen as being comparable to the top of a real desk in an actual office or den. Starting a program is like taking a folder full of papers out of storage and placing it on the desk. To do some work in the real world, of course, you need to pull papers out of a folder and place them on the desk. This is just like opening a file within the program (it could be a letter, a drawing, an email message, or whatever). To extend the metaphor a little, most programs also come with tools, such as a ruler, a calculator, and a calendar, that are the electronic equivalents of the tools you use at your desk.

So officially, the vast expanse that takes up the bulk of the screen real estate is the Windows desktop, and it's where you'll do your work.

The Taskbar

The strip along the bottom of the Windows screen is called the *taskbar*. The taskbar sports four distinct features (pointed out in Figure 2.2).

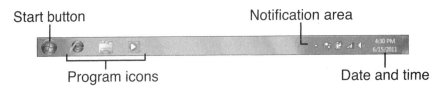

Figure 2.2: The features of the Windows 7 taskbar.

- **Start button.** Believe it or not, this tiny chunk of screen is one of the most important features in all of Windows. As its name implies, the Start button is your starting point for most of the Windows features and goodies. I discuss the Start button in depth in Chapter 3.

- **Program icons.** This area contains a few icons. An *icon* is a small picture that represents something on your system, such as a program or a command. You use these icons to start programs and to control running programs, as I natter on about in Chapter 3.

- **Notification area.** Windows uses this area to let you know when something important (or at least, something that Windows *thinks* is important) is happening with your machine. These are called *notifications*, and they'll pop up from time to time to keep you in the know.

- **Date and time.** This area's purpose is obvious enough: it tells you the current date and time.

A Few Mouse and Keyboard Fundamentals

Okay, if Windows is supposed to have all kinds of fancy-schmancy features, how do you get at them? Ah, that's where your mouse and keyboard come in. You use them as "input devices" to give Windows its marching orders. If you're new to computers, the next few sections show you the basic mouse and keyboard techniques you need to know.

Basic Mouse Maneuvers

If you're unfamiliar with Windows, there's a good chance that you're also unfamiliar with the mouse—the electromechanical (and thankfully, toothless) mammal attached to your machine. If so, this section presents a quick look at a few mouse moves, which is important because much of what you do in Windows will involve the mouse in some way.

For starters, be sure the mouse is sitting on its pad or on your desk with the cord facing away from you. (If you have one of those newfangled cordless mice, move the mouse so that the buttons are facing away from you.) Rest your hand lightly on the mouse with your index finger on (but not pressing down) the left button and your middle finger on the right button (or the rightmost button). Southpaws need to reverse the fingering.

Figure 2.1, displayed earlier, showed you the *mouse pointer*. Find the pointer on your screen, then slowly move the mouse on its pad. As you do this, notice that the pointer moves in the same direction. Take a few minutes to practice moving the pointer to and fro, using slow, easy movements. (Don't be alarmed if the mouse pointer stops dead in its tracks when it reaches the edge of the screen. This is perfectly normal behavior, and you can get the pointer going again by moving the mouse in the opposite direction.)

The secret to mastering the mouse is threefold. First, use the same advice as was given to the person who wanted to get to Carnegie Hall: practice, practice, practice. Fortunately, with Windows being so mouse-dependent, you'll get plenty of chances to perfect your skills. Second, configure the mouse to allow for any dexterity challenges you might have. I show you how to do this in Chapter 9. Third, understand all the basic mouse moves that are required of the modern-day mouse user. There are a half-dozen in all:

- **Point**. Move the mouse pointer so that it's positioned over some specified part of the screen. For example, "point at the Start button" means that you move the mouse pointer over the taskbar's Start button.

- **Click**. Press and immediately release the left mouse button to initiate some kind of action. Need a "fer instance"? Okay, point at the Start button and then click it. Instantly, a menu pops up in response to the click. (This is Windows' Start menu. I'll discuss it in detail in Chapter 3. For now, you can get rid of the menu either by clicking an empty section of the desktop or by pressing the **Esc** key on your keyboard.)

- **Double-click**. Press and release the left mouse button *twice*, one press right after the other (there should be little or no delay between each press). To give it a whirl, point at the desktop's Recycle Bin icon and then double-click. If all goes well, Windows will toss a box titled Recycle Bin onto the desktop. To return this box from whence it came, click the **X** button in the upper-right corner. If nothing happens when you double-click, try to click as quickly as you can—and try not to move the mouse while you're clicking.

> **By the Way**
>
> Okay, so clicking initiates some kind of action, but so does double-clicking. What's the diff? The entire single-click versus double-click conundrum is one of the most confusing and criticized traits in Windows, and I'm afraid there's no easy answer. Just know that some things require just a click to get going, whereas other things require a double-click. With experience, you'll eventually come to know which clicking technique is needed.

- **Right-click**. Press and immediately release the *right* mouse button. In Windows, the right-click is used almost exclusively to display the *shortcut menu*. To see one, right-click an empty part of the desktop. Windows displays a menu with a few common commands related to the desktop. To remove this menu, *left*-click the desktop.

- **Click and drag.** Point at some object, press and *hold down* the left mouse button, move the mouse, and then release the button. You almost always use this technique to move an object from one place to another. For example, try dragging the desktop's Recycle Bin icon. (To restore apple-pie order to the desktop, right-click the desktop, click **Sort By** in the shortcut menu, and then click **Name**.)

- **Scroll.** This means that you turn the little wheel that's nestled between the left and right mouse buttons. In programs that support scrolling, you use this technique to move up and down within a document. The wheel is a relatively new innovation, so your mouse may not have one. If not, never fear—because Windows provides other ways to navigate a document, as you'll see in Chapter 4.

Common Keyboard Conveniences

I mentioned earlier that getting comfy with your mouse is crucial if you want to make your Windows life as easy as possible. That's not to say, however, that the keyboard never comes in handy as a timesaver. On the contrary, Windows is chock-full of keyboard shortcuts that are sometimes quicker than standard mouse techniques. I'll tell you about these shortcuts as we go along. For now, let's run through some of the standard keyboard parts and see how they fit into the Windows way of doing things:

- **The Ctrl and Alt keys.** If you press **Ctrl** (it's pronounced "control") or **Alt** (it's pronounced "alt" as in *alt*ernate), nothing much happens—but that's okay, because nothing much is supposed to happen. You don't use these keys by themselves but as part of *key combinations*. (The **Shift** key often gets into the act as well.) For example, hold down the **Ctrl** key with one hand, use your other hand to tap the **Esc** key, and then release **Ctrl**. Like magic, you see a menu of options sprout from the Start button. (To hide this menu again, press **Esc** by itself.)

Definition

A **key combination** is a keyboard technique where you hold down one key and then press another key (or possibly two other keys).

- **The Esc key.** Your keyboard's Esc (or Escape) key is your all-purpose, get-me-the-heck-out-of-here key. For example, you just saw that you can get rid of the Start menu by pressing **Esc**. In many cases, if you do something in Windows that you didn't want to do, you can reverse your tracks with a quick tap (or maybe two or three) of **Esc**.

- **The numeric keypad.** On a standard keyboard layout, the numeric keypad is the separate collection of numbered keys on the right. The numeric keypad usually serves two functions, and you toggle between these functions by pressing the **Num Lock** key. (Most keyboards have a Num Lock indicator light that tells you when the Num Lock is on.) When the Num Lock is on, you can use the numeric keypad to type numbers. When the Num Lock is off, the other symbols on the keys become active. For example, the **8** key's upward-pointing arrow becomes active, which means you can use it to move up within a program. Some keyboards (called *extended keyboards*) have a separate keypad for the insertion-point movement keys, and you can keep Num Lock on all the time.

> **Good to Know!**
> Let's put the mouse and keyboard to work to determine which version of Windows you're using. Click the **Start** button, click **Computer** (or **My Computer**), press **Alt+H** to display the Help menu, and then click **About Windows**. The window that appears will tell you which version of Windows you're running.

Windows' keyboard combo shortcuts pop up regularly throughout the book. Because I'm *way* too lazy to write out something like, "Hold down the **Ctrl** key with one hand, use your other hand to tap the **Esc** key, and then release **Ctrl**" each time, I use the following shorthand notation instead: "Press **Hold+Tap**," where **Hold** is the key you hold down and **Tap** is the key you tap. In other words, "Press **Ctrl+Esc**." (On rare occasions, a third key joins the parade, so you may see something like, "Press **Ctrl+Alt+Delete**." In this case, you hold down the first two keys and then tap the third key.)

Shutting Down and Restarting Your Computer

When you've stood just about all you can stand of your computer for one day, it's time to close up shop. Please tape the following to your cat's forehead so that you never forget it: *Never, I repeat, never turn off your computer's power while Windows is still running.* Doing so can lead to data loss, a trashed configuration, and accelerated hair loss that those new pills don't help.

Putting Your Computer to Sleep

Now that I've scared the daylights out of you, let's learn the proper procedure for shutting down your computer. First, note that the steps I'm going to show you will put your computer to sleep. This means that Windows not only shuts down your computer but also "remembers" which windows and programs you have running. When you restart Windows, it restores those programs and windows automatically, which is very handy.

Follow these steps to put your computer to sleep:

1. Click the **Start** button to pop up the Start menu.

2. Click the arrow to the right of the **Shut down** button. This pops up another menu, as shown in Figure 2.3.

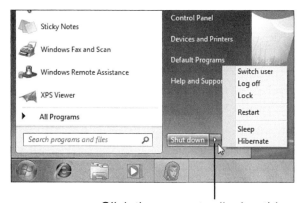

Click the arrow to display this menu.

Figure 2.3: Click the arrow to the right of the Shut down button to see this menu.

3. Click **Sleep**. Windows dutifully tucks in your computer for the night.

If you're using Windows Vista, you put your computer to sleep by clicking **Start** and then clicking the **Sleep** button (it's to the left of the button that has a Lock icon on it). If you're using Windows XP, you put your computer to sleep by clicking **Start**, clicking **Turn Off Computer**, and then clicking **Stand By**.

Restarting Your Computer

Rather than putting your computer to sleep, there will be times when you shut down and then immediately restart your computer. Why on earth would you want to do such a thing? The most common reason is to fix a problem with your computer. For example, if you find that a program is crashing frequently, restarting can often make things right.

Follow these steps to restart your computer:

1. Click the **Start** button to pop up the Start menu.
2. Click the arrow to the right of the **Shut down** button.
3. Click **Restart**. Windows shuts down and then restarts your computer.

If you're using Windows Vista, you restart your computer by clicking **Start**, clicking the arrow to the right of the button that has a Lock icon on it, and then clicking **Restart**. If you're using Windows XP, restart your computer by clicking **Start**, clicking **Turn Off Computer**, and then clicking **Restart**.

The Least You Need to Know

- The Windows 7 screen is carved into two main areas: the desktop—the large area that covers most of your monitor—and the taskbar—the thin strip along the bottom of the screen.
- The three most-used mouse movements are the click (quickly pressing and releasing the left mouse button), the double-click (two quick clicks), and the click and drag (holding down the left button and moving the mouse).
- A key combination involves holding down one key, pressing a second key, and then releasing the first key.
- To put your computer to sleep, click **Start**, click the arrow, and then click **Sleep**.

Installing and Running Programs

Chapter 3

In This Chapter

- Installing software
- Uninstalling programs you no longer need
- Using the Start menu to launch a program
- Learning about pull-down menus, toolbars, and dialog boxes
- Techniques for switching between programs
- Shutting down a program

If you want to get your computer to do anything even remotely non-paperweight–like, you need to launch and work with a program or three. For example, if you want to write a memo or a letter, you need to fire up a word-processing program; if you want to draw pictures, you need to crank up a graphics program. If you want to use the Windows spreadsheet program, well … there isn't one. Windows 7 comes with a passel of programs, but a spreadsheet isn't among them. If you want to crunch numbers, you need to get a third-party spreadsheet program, such as Microsoft Excel.

On the other hand, Windows 7 *does* come with a decent collection of programs that enable you to perform most run-of-the-mill computing tasks. This chapter shows you how to get at those programs as well as how to mess with them after they're up and running.

Installing a Program

It's one thing to understand that the computer is a versatile beast that can handle all kinds of different programs, but it's quite another to actually install the stuff. The first half of this chapter will help by showing you exactly how to install software programs—and for good measure, how to uninstall them—just in case they don't get along with your computer or you find you don't need them.

Installing Windows Live Essentials Programs

Windows Live Essentials is a collection of free programs that Microsoft makes available on the internet for downloading to your computer. These programs include Windows Live Mail (for working with email; see Chapter 12) and Windows Live Photo Gallery (for viewing and editing digital photos; see Chapter 5).

To get your mitts on these programs, you need to connect to the internet (as explained in Chapter 10), download them, and then install them. Fortunately, Windows Live uses an installation program to handle most of the dirty work for you automatically, so you need only follow these steps:

1. Click the **Start** button, click **Getting Started**, and then double-click **Go online to get Windows Live Essentials**. Internet Explorer opens and heads for the Windows Live Essentials page. (If this is the first you've seen any of this Internet Explorer business, see Chapter 11 for a crash course.)

By the Way

If you don't see the Getting Started command anywhere, not to worry. Start Internet Explorer yourself and surf to the following address: http://download.live.com. You can also use this address to install Windows Live Essentials on Windows Vista. Sadly, the Windows Live Essentials programs don't run on Windows XP.

2. Click **Download now**. Internet Explorer displays the File Download—Security Warning dialog box. (I'll explain what dialog boxes are later in this chapter, in the aptly titled section, "Dialog Boxes.")

3. Click **Run**. Now you're pestered by the User Account Control dialog box, which asks for your permission to install a program.

4. Click **Yes**. Windows Live thinks about things for a while, then displays the What Do You Want to Install? screen.

5. Click **Choose the programs you want to install**. You then come face-to-face with the Select Programs to Install screen, shown in Figure 3.1.

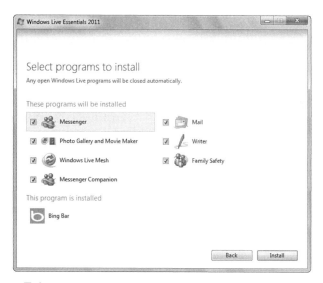

Figure 3.1: Use this window to decide which Windows Live Essentials programs you want to shoehorn into your PC.

6. Click to remove the check mark next to each program you don't want to install. (If you're not sure about a particular program, point at it with your mouse to see a description.)

7. Click **Install**. Windows Live installs your selected programs.

Installing a New Program

The built-in Windows programs (and the not-quite-built-in Windows Live Essentials programs) do the job as long as your needs aren't too lofty. However, what if your needs *are* lofty or you're looking to fill in a software niche that Windows doesn't cover (such as a spreadsheet program, a database, or a game)? In that case, you need to go outside the Windows box (literally!) and purchase the appropriate program. (This often means going to a computer store, but you can also purchase software over the internet.)

After you have the program, your next task is to install it. This means you run a "setup" routine that makes the program ready for use on your computer. How you launch this setup routine depends on how the program is distributed:

- **If the program is on a disc:** After you insert the disc, Windows automatically looks for an installation program. If it finds one, it displays the AutoPlay box with an option that says something like, "Run SETUP.EXE" (see Figure 3.2). Click that option to get the installation under way.

- **If you purchased the program on the internet:** In this case, the vendor will supply you with a "Download" link to get the installation file onto your computer. When you click that link, Internet Explorer will ask what you want to do with the file (see Figure 3.3), and your best bet here is to click **Run**. This brings the file to your computer and starts the installation.

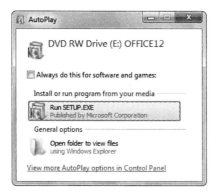

Figure 3.2: When you insert a program's installation disc, Windows displays the AutoPlay box on the screen, and you then click Run SETUP.EXE (or something similar).

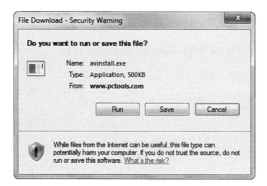

Figure 3.3: When Internet Explorer asks what you want to do with the file, click **Run** for fastest service.

From here, follow the instructions and prompts that the setup routine gives you. (This procedure varies from program to program.)

Uninstalling a Program

Most programs seem like good ideas at the time you install them. Unless you're an outright pessimist, you probably figured that a program you installed was going to help you work harder, be more efficient, or have more fun. Sadly, many programs don't live up to expectations. The good news is that you don't have to put up with a loser program after you realize it's not up to snuff. You can *uninstall* it so that it doesn't clutter up your Start menu, desktop, hard disk, or any other location where it might have insinuated itself.

> **Definition**
>
> When you **uninstall** a program, you completely remove that program from your computer.

Uninstalling a Windows Live Essentials Program

Okay, so you installed Windows Live Mesh and Family Safety from Windows Live and you *still* don't know what the heck they do. No problem! You can ditch them and any other Windows Live Essential program you don't need. Here's how:

1. Select **Start**, **Control Panel** to launch Control Panel.

2. Under the **Programs** heading, click **Uninstall a program**. Windows 7 displays a list of the programs installed on your computer.

3. In the list of programs, click **Windows Live Essentials**. If you don't see it, click any program in the list and then press **W** until Windows Live Essentials is highlighted.

4. Click the **Uninstall/Change** button. The Uninstall or Repair Windows Live Programs window appears.

5. Click **Remove one or more Windows Live programs**. Windows Live displays a list of the Essentials programs taking up space on your computer.

6. Activate the check box beside each program you want to throw out.

7. Click **Uninstall**. Windows Live removes the programs, and a few minutes later it asks you to restart your computer.

8. Click **Restart Now**. If you're busy with something and don't want to restart, that's okay. Click **Restart Later** instead, finish your business, and then restart your computer when you're done.

Giving a Program the Heave-Ho

If you have a Windows application that has worn out its welcome, this section shows you a couple methods for uninstalling the darn thing so that it's out of your life forever. The good news is that Windows 7 has a feature that enables you to remove any application with a simple mouse click. The bad news is that this feature is only available for some programs.

To check whether it's available for your program, follow these steps:

1. Select **Start**, **Control Panel** to launch the Control Panel.

2. Under **Programs**, click the **Uninstall a program** link. Windows 7 displays a list of the programs installed on your computer.

3. Click the program you want to remove.

4. Click the **Uninstall** button (or it may be called **Uninstall/Change**).

5. What happens next depends on the program. You may see a dialog box asking you to confirm the uninstall, or you may be asked whether you want to run an "Automatic" or "Custom" uninstall. For the latter, be sure to select the **Automatic** option. Whatever happens, follow the instructions on the screen until you return to the Add or Remove Programs window.

Good to Know!

Don't be surprised if the uninstall routine doesn't wipe out absolutely everything for a program. For example, if you created any documents using the program, the uninstall program politely leaves them on your system just in case you need them.

Launching a Program

If you're interested in starting a program, then you might think the Start button in the lower-left corner of the screen would be a promising place to begin. If so, give yourself a pat on the back—because that's exactly right. Go ahead and use your mouse to point at the Start button, then click. As you can see in Figure 3.4, Windows responds by displaying a rather large box on the screen. This is called the *Start menu*, and you'll be visiting this particular place a lot in your Windows travels.

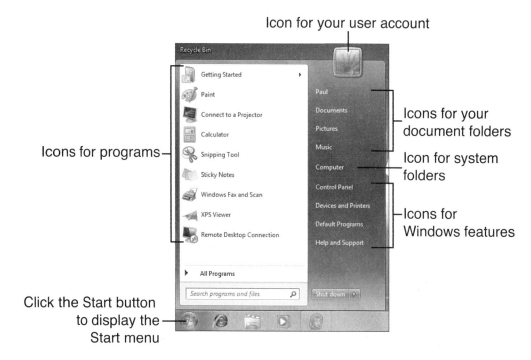

Figure 3.4: The Start menu.

A Look at the Start Menu

The Start menu is populated with all kinds of icons. An *icon* is a picture representing something that exists on your computer. To see what I mean, let's run through the various icons that exist on the Start menu. (Again, however, I need to point out that computer manufacturers can and will customize the Start menu, so yours may be populated with a different set of icons.) As pointed out in Figure 3.4, I divide the icons into four general categories: programs, document folders, system folders, and Windows features.

For the programs, the initial Start menu has a few icons for applications such as Paint (for drawing stuff on your computer) and Calculator (for simple number crunching).

More importantly for our purposes, Windows 7's standard-issue Start menu includes a program called Getting Started, which has a few more icons for tasks related to folks who are just getting acquainted with Windows 7. We'll tackle many of those tasks throughout the book, but for now I want you to puzzle over the teensy little arrow that appears to the right of the Getting Started icon. If you position the mouse pointer over that arrow, the Start menu transforms itself into the version you see in Figure 3.5. Now, the right side of the menu displays a collection of smaller, cuter icons under the heading Tasks. This is called a *jump list*, and basically it's a list of tasks associated with a particular program. You click a task to run it. (To send the jump list back from whence it came, press **Esc**.)

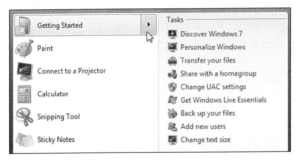

Figure 3.5: Move your mouse pointer over the little arrow to see a program's jump list (if it has one).

The document folders section of the Start menu is populated with four icons:

- **User name**. This icon represents the main *folder* assigned to your Windows user account, and it is given the same name as your user account (for example, Paul). This folder contains all your *documents*.

Definition

A **folder** is a storage location on your computer's hard disk. What do you store in a folder? You store files, which generally come in two flavors: **documents** that you create yourself and program files that run the programs installed on your computer.

- **Documents**. This icon represents the folder where you'll store most of the documents that you create. (You'll learn what it's all about in Chapter 4.)
- **Pictures**. This icon represents the folder where you'll store your picture files (which are also known as graphics files and image files; see Chapter 5 for more information).
- **Music**. This icon represents the folder where you'll store your music files, as described in Chapter 5.

The system folders part of the Start menu is populated with just one icon: Computer. This icon represents the folder that contains everything on your computer, including your hard disk, CD or DVD drive, and removable drives.

For the Windows 7 features, the Start menu is home to four icons:

- **Control Panel**. This icon represents the Windows Control Panel feature, which you use to customize Windows. I talk about the Control Panel throughout this book.

- **Devices and Printers**. This icon opens a window that shows you all the major devices that are attached to your computer.

- **Default Programs**. This icon represents a program that you can use to customize the programs that Windows uses for certain actions, such as browsing the internet.

- **Help and Support**. This icon represents the Windows Help feature, which offers guidance and instruction on Windows' various bits and pieces.

Finally, the Start menu has two other features that you need to know:

- **All Programs**. This icon represents another menu that lists all the other programs installed on your computer. (See the next section, "Navigating the Start Menu," to learn more about this icon.)

- **Search programs and files**. This doohickey isn't an icon at all but what's known in the Windows trade as a *text box*—so-called because you use it to type text. In this case, you type a word or two related to something you want to find on your computer, and Windows displays icons for everything on your system that matches your typing. It all sounds quite mysterious, I know, but you'll get the full scoop in Chapter 4.

Navigating the Start Menu

Now that you've met the denizens of the Start menu, you need to know how to make them do something useful. To launch an icon, you have two possibilities:

- For every icon except All Programs, you need only click the icon and Windows 7 launches the program, folder, or feature without further ado.

- Clicking the **All Programs** icon brings up another menu, as shown in Figure 3.6. As you can see, this new menu is filled with even more icons. To launch one of these icons, click it with your mouse.

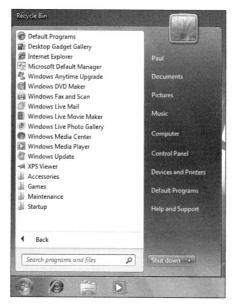

Figure 3.6: Clicking the **All Programs** icon displays a menu of programs.

Notice, however, that the icons at the bottom (Accessories, Games, and so on) have a folder icon to the left. When you click one of these icons, a new menu (called a *submenu*) slides out below the icon. For example, clicking the Accessories icon displays the submenu shown in Figure 3.7.

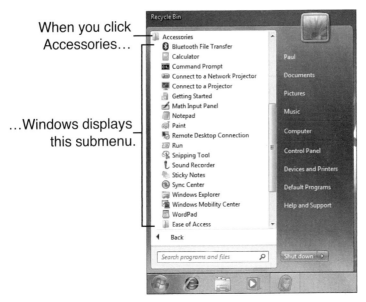

Figure 3.7: Some icons exist only to display a submenu that contains even more icons.

Don't be surprised if you find yourself wading through two or three of these submenus to get the program you want. For example, here are the steps you'd follow to fire up Magnifier, the program you use to magnify hard-to-see parts of the screen (see Chapter 7):

1. Click the **Start** button to display the Start menu.

2. Click **All Programs** to open the menu.

3. Click **Accessories** to open the submenu.

4. Click **Ease of Access** to open yet another submenu.

5. Click **Magnifier**. Windows 7 launches the Disk Cleanup program. (If you follow these steps but don't actually want to use Magnifier right now, click the **X** that appears in the upper-right corner of the screen.)

In the future, I abbreviate these long-winded Start menu procedures by using a comma (,) to separate each item you click, like so: "Select **Start, All Programs, Accessories, Ease of Access, Magnifier**."

> **Good to Know!**
>
> In Windows 7, you get another way to fire up programs. Take a peek at the Windows 7 taskbar, particularly the three icons to the right of the Start button. These icons represent three programs—Internet Explorer, Windows Explorer, and Windows Media Player—and all it takes is a single click from you and the associated program launches without any further fuss. How easy is *that?*

Working with Programs

Okay, so you know how to get a program running. What's next? Now you get to go on a little personal power trip, because this section shows you how to boss around your programs. Specifically, you learn how to work with pull-down menus, toolbars, and dialog boxes.

Pull-Down Menus

Each program you work with has a set of commands and features that define the majority of what you can do with the program. Most of these commands and features are available via the program's *pull-down menus*. Oh sure, there are easier ways to tell a program what to do (I talk about some of them later in this chapter), but pull-down menus are special because they offer a complete road map for any program.

I'm going to use the Windows Explorer program as an example for the next page or two. If you feel like following along, go ahead and launch the program by clicking the **Windows Explorer** icon on the taskbar. (If you've grown inordinately fond of the Start menu, you can also click **Start** and then click your user icon.)

The first thing you need to know is that a program's pull-down menus are housed in the *menu bar*, the horizontal strip that runs across the window, as pointed out in Figure 3.8. Note that in Windows Explorer, you need to press the **Alt** key to display the menu bar. (Most programs display the menu bar automatically.) Each word in the menu bar represents a pull-down menu.

Good to Know!

If I didn't know better, I'd swear that Windows 7 is a bit embarrassed to be seen with its pull-down menus. That's because many Windows 7 programs operate with the menu bar hidden away like some crazy aunt. If you open a program and don't see the menus, pressing the **Alt** key should bring the menu bar into the light of day.

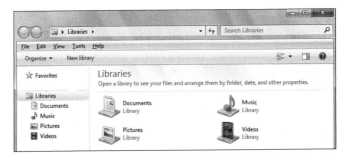

Figure 3.8: In Windows Explorer, press **Alt** to display the menu bar.

The various items that run across the menu bar (such as File, Edit, and View in Windows Explorer) are the names of the menus. To see (that is, *pull down*) one of these menus, use your mouse to click the menu name. For example, click **View** to pull down the View menu, as shown in Figure 3.9.

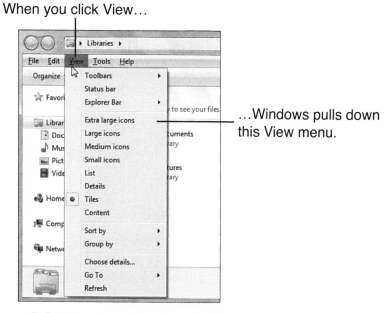

Figure 3.9: Windows Explorer's View menu.

The various items you see in the menu are called *commands*. From here, use your mouse to click the command you want.

Definition

A **command** is a menu item that initiates some kind of action.

Throughout this book, I tell you to select a pull-down menu command by separating the menu name and command name with a comma (,): "Select the **View, Refresh** command."

What happens next depends on which command you picked. (What if you don't want to choose a command? No sweat: press **Alt** to get rid of the menu.) Here's a summary of the various possibilities.

- **The command runs without further fuss.** This is the simplest scenario, and it just means that the program carries out the command—no questions asked. For example, clicking the **View** menu's **Refresh** command updates Windows Explorer's display automatically.

- **Another menu appears.** As shown in Figure 3.10, when you click the **View** menu's **Sort By** command, a submenu appears on the right. You then click the command you want to execute from the new menu.

- **The command is toggled on or off.** Some commands operate like light switches: they toggle certain features of a program on and off. When the feature is on, a small check mark appears to the left of the command to let you know. Selecting the command turns off the feature and removes the check mark. If you select the command again, the feature turns back on and the check mark reappears. For example, click the **View** menu's **Status Bar** command, which activates the status bar at the bottom of the Windows Explorer window (see Figure 3.10).

- **An option is activated.** Besides having features that you can toggle on and off, some programs have flexible features that can assume three or more different states. Windows Explorer, for example, gives you eight ways to display the contents of your computer, according to your choice of one of the following View menu commands: **Extra Large Icons**, **Large Icons**, **Medium Icons**, **Small Icons**, **List**, **Details**, **Tiles**, and **Content**. Because these states are mutually exclusive (you can select only one at a time), you need some way of knowing which of the eight commands is currently active. That's the job of the *option mark:* a small dot that appears to the left of the active command (see the Tiles command in Figure 3.10).

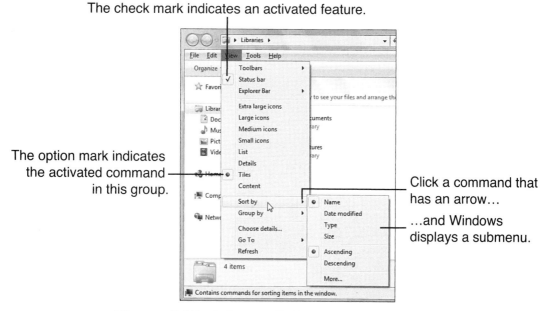

Figure 3.10: A few pull-down menu features.

- **A dialog box appears**. Dialog boxes are little windows that show up whenever the program needs to ask you for more information. You learn more about them in the "Dialog Boxes" section later in this chapter.

Toolbars

The computer wizards who build our programs have come up with some amazing things over the years, but one of their most useful inventions has to be the *toolbar*. This is a collection of easily accessible icons designed to give you push-button access to common commands and features. There are no unsightly key combinations to remember and no pull-down menu forests to get lost in.

Toolbars play a big role in Windows, and you can reap some big dividends if you get to know how they work.

In Windows Explorer, the toolbar is the horizontal strip that sits just below the menu bar (when it's displayed, that is). This is actually a special type of toolbar called a *taskbar*, because what you see on the toolbar is really a collection of tasks you can perform for whatever item you're working on within the window. No matter: it still works like most toolbars, so it will serve us well as an example.

Most toolbar icons are buttons that represent commands you'd normally access by using the pull-down menus. All you have to do is click a button, and the program runs the command. However, you'll occasionally come across toolbar buttons that are really pull-down-menu wannabes. In Windows Explorer, the Organize "button" is an example of this species. As shown in Figure 3.11, the button has a downward-pointing arrow, which means that when you click the button you see a list of commands or options.

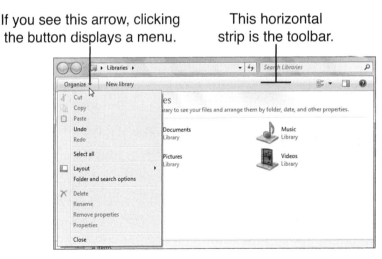

Figure 3.11: Like most Windows programs, Windows Explorer comes with a toolbar.

Special Cases: WordPad, Paint, and Windows Live

Just to confuse the issue, two of the programs you may end up using fairly often have completely different (and potentially baffling) ways to run commands. These programs are WordPad (a word processor), Paint (a graphics program), and most of the Windows Live programs I mentioned earlier (such as Windows Live Mail and Windows Live Photo Gallery).

To see what I'm talking about, go ahead and get WordPad onto the desktop by selecting **Start**, **All Programs**, **Accessories**, **WordPad**. As you can see in Figure 3.12, WordPad is weird in two ways: there's no menu bar (and you can tap **Alt** until your finger falls off), and the toolbar is *huge*. Actually, that's not a toolbar at all but something called a *ribbon*, which is kind of like a toolbar on steroids.

By the Way

None of the programs that come with Windows Vista or Windows XP use the ribbon. You'll only see the ribbon in Vista if you install any of the "ribbonized" Windows Live programs.

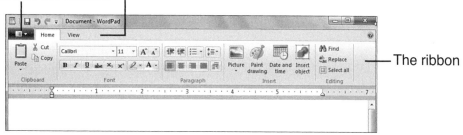

Figure 3.12: In Windows 7, WordPad (as well as Paint and some Windows Live programs) comes with a new-fangled ribbon for faster access to program features.

The ribbon works basically the same as a regular toolbar, with the major difference being the presence of two tabs: Home and View. (Other ribbon-enhanced programs may have more tabs.) Click these tabs to see more buttons. Also, to get to the program's menus, you need to click the button in the upper-left corner that I point out in Figure 3.12.

Dialog Boxes

I mentioned earlier that after you select some menu commands, the program may require more information from you. For example, if you run a Print command, the program may want to know how many copies of the document you want to print.

In these situations, the program sends an emissary to parley with you. These emissaries, called *dialog boxes*, are one of the most ubiquitous features in the Windows world. This section preps you for your dialog box conversations by showing you how to work with every type of dialog box control you're likely to encounter. (They're called *controls* because you use them to manipulate the different dialog box settings.) Before starting, it's important to keep in mind that most dialog boxes like to monopolize your attention. When one is on the screen, you usually can't do anything else in the program (such as select a pull-down menu). Deal with the dialog box first, and then you can move on to other things.

Definition

A **dialog box** is a small window that a program uses to prompt you for information or to display a message. You interact with each dialog box by using one or more **controls** to input data or initiate actions.

Okay, let's get started. Please refer to Figure 3.13 for examples of the following dialog box controls:

- **Command button**. Clicking one of these buttons executes whatever command is written on the button. The two examples shown in Figure 3.13 are the most common. You click **OK** to close the dialog box and put the settings into effect, or you click **Cancel** to close the dialog box without doing anything. In many dialog boxes, you can also click **Help** to view the program's Help system.

- **Check box**. Windows uses a check box to toggle program features on and off. Clicking the check box either adds a check mark (meaning the feature will get turned on when you click **OK**) or removes the check mark (meaning the feature will get turned off when you click **OK**).

- **Option button**. If a program feature offers two or more mutually exclusive possibilities, the dialog box will offer an option button for each state, and only one button can be activated (that is, have a blue dot inside its circle) at a time. You activate an option button by clicking it.

- **Drop-down list box**. This control contains a list of items. In this case, at first you see only one item. However, if you click the downward-pointing arrow on the right, the full list appears and you can click the item you want.

- **Text box**. You use this control to type text data.

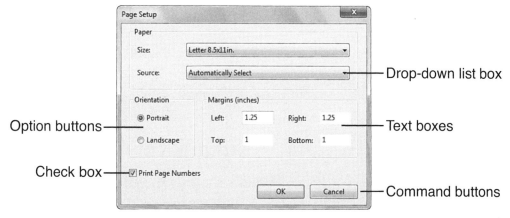

Figure 3.13: This dialog box demonstrates quite a few dialog box features.

Please refer to Figure 3.14 for examples of the following dialog box controls:

- **Tab**. Click any of the tabs displayed across the top of some dialog boxes, and you'll see a new set of controls.
- **List box**. These controls display a list of items, and you select an item by clicking it.
- **Slider**. Click and drag the slider to set the value of the control.

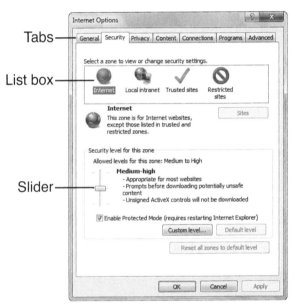

Figure 3.14: A few more dialog box controls to make your day.

Switching from One Program to Another

When you fire up a program, Windows marks the occasion by adding a button to the taskbar. If you then add another program or two onto the screen (remember, Windows is capable of *multitasking*—running multiple programs simultaneously), each one gets its own taskbar button.

For example, Figure 3.15 shows Windows with two programs up and running: WordPad and Paint. (To run the latter, select **Start**, **All Programs**, **Accessories**, **Paint**.) It looks as though Paint has lopped off a good portion of the WordPad window, but in reality Windows is just displaying Paint "on top" of WordPad. Also notice that in the taskbar there are now buttons for both WordPad and Paint.

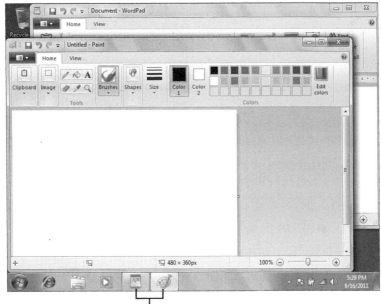

Each running program gets its own taskbar button.

Figure 3.15: Windows with two programs running.

The taskbar has another trick up its digital sleeve: you can switch from one running program to another by clicking the latter's taskbar button. For example, when I click the WordPad button, the WordPad window comes forward, as shown in Figure 3.16.

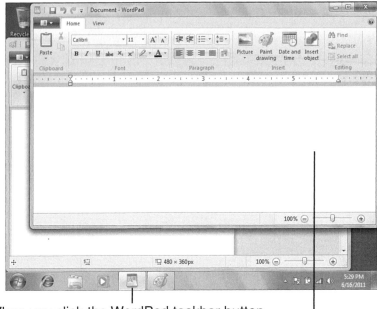

When you click the WordPad taskbar button…

…the WordPad window elbows its way to the front.

Figure 3.16: You can use the taskbar buttons to switch from one program to another.

Besides clicking the taskbar buttons, you can also leap from one running program to another by clicking the program's window. This is perhaps the simplest and most obvious method because all you do is point the mouse inside the program's window and then click. This method is most useful if your hand is already on the mouse and you can see at least part of the window you want to activate.

Quitting a Program

When you're finished with a particular program, you should close it to keep your screen uncluttered and to reduce the load on Windows' resources. The easiest way is to click the **Close** button—the "X" in the upper-right corner of the program's window. You can also pull down the program's **File** menu and select the **Exit** command (or, more rarely, the **Close** command).

Depending on the program you're closing and the work you were doing with it, you may be asked whether you want to save some files. Be sure to click **Yes** (or **OK** or **Save** or whatever command actually saves your work). You'll learn lots more about saving files in Chapter 4.

The Least You Need to Know

- Most software discs support AutoPlay, so the installation program runs automatically after you insert the disc.
- To start a program, click the **Start** button to display the Start menu, then click the command or submenus required to launch the program.
- To select a pull-down menu command, first display the menu by clicking its name in the menu bar, and then click the command.
- In a dialog box, click **OK** to put dialog box settings into effect; click **Cancel** to bail out of a dialog box without doing anything; or click **Help** to view the program's Help system.
- To switch between running programs, click the taskbar buttons. Alternatively, click the program window if you can see a chunk of it.
- To quit a program, click the **Close** (X) button. You can also usually get away with selecting the program's **File**, **Exit** command.

Chapter 4

Dealing with Documents

In This Chapter

- Defining a document
- Forging a fresh document
- Basic document-editing techniques
- Saving a document for posterity
- Closing a document and opening it again
- Using libraries and folders to organize your documents
- Locating a document in even the messiest hard drive

The purpose of the chapters in Part 1 is to help you get comfortable with your computer, and if you've been following along and practicing what you've learned, you and your new digital friend should be getting along famously by now. However, there's another concept you need to familiarize yourself with before you're ready to fully explore the computing universe: documents.

This chapter plugs that gap in your computer education by teaching you all the basic Windows techniques for manipulating documents. This includes creating, saving, editing, closing, finding, and opening documents—plus much more.

What Is a Document?

In the real world, a *document* is a letter, a memo, a brochure, or really, anything that has text on it (and perhaps a picture or two). So from the previous chapter, you may be tempted to think that a computer document is a word-processing file. After all, you can use a word-processing program to create a letter, a memo, a brochure, and so on.

That's certainly true, but I'm talking about a bigger picture in this chapter. Specifically, when I say "document," what I really mean is *any* file that you create yourself, or that someone else has created, by working with a software program.

So yes, a file created within the confines of a word-processing program (such as WordPad) is a document. However, these are also documents: text notes you type into a text editor, images you draw in a graphics program, email missives you compose in an email program, spreadsheets you construct with a spreadsheet program, and presentations you cobble together with a graphics presentation program. In other words, if you can create it or edit it yourself, it's a document.

Creating a New Document

Lots of Windows programs—including WordPad, Notepad, and Paint—are courteous enough to offer a new, ready-to-roll document when you start the program. This means you can just dive right in to your typing, drawing, or whatever. Later, however, you may need to create another new document. To do so, use one of the following techniques:

- Select the **File, New** command. In WordPad (select **Start, All Programs, Accessories, WordPad**), which doesn't have a menu bar, click the **WordPad** button (pointed out in Figure 4.1; a similar button appears in Paint and in the Microsoft Office programs, such as Word and Excel) to open the new style of File menu, then click **New**.

- Click the **New** button in the program's toolbar.

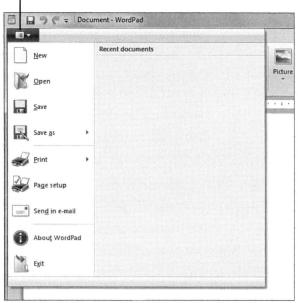

Figure 4.1: You usually start a new document by displaying the File menu and selecting the New command.

- In many Windows programs, you can crank out a new document by pressing **Ctrl+N**.

Entering and Editing Document Text

As you work with a document, you have to delete text, move text to different locations, and so on. To make your electronic writing life easier, it's crucial to get these basic editing chores down pat. To that end, here's a summary of some editing techniques you can use in most any program that deals with text (including Notepad, WordPad, and Windows Live Mail):

- **Highlighting text with the mouse** Before you can do something to existing text, you need to *highlight* it. To highlight text with a mouse, click and drag the mouse over the characters you want. That is, you first position the mouse pointer a teensy bit to the left of the first character you want to highlight. Then, you press and hold down the left mouse button and move the mouse to the right. As you do, the characters you pass over become highlighted. While you drag, you can also move the mouse down to highlight multiple lines. When you release the mouse button, the text remains highlighted.

- **Highlighting text with the keyboard** To highlight text by using the keyboard, position the cursor to the left of the first character, hold down the **Shift** key, and then press the **right-arrow** key until the entire selection is highlighted. Use the **down-arrow** key (or even **Page Down** if you have a lot of ground to cover) when you need to highlight multiple lines.

What Can Go Wrong?

If you highlight some text and then press a character on your keyboard, your entire selection will disappear and be replaced by the character you typed! (If you press the **Enter** key, the highlighted text just disappears entirely.) This is normal behavior that can cause trouble for even experienced document jockeys. To restore your text, immediately select the **Edit**, **Undo** command or press **Ctrl+Z**.

- **Copying and pasting highlighted text**   To make a copy of the highlighted text, select the **Edit**, **Copy** command. (Alternatively, you can also press **Ctrl+C** or click the **Copy** toolbar button.) Then, position the cursor where you want to place the copy and select the **Edit**, **Paste** command. (Your other choices are to press **Ctrl+V** or click the **Paste** toolbar button.) A perfect copy of your selection appears instantly. Note that you can paste this text as many times as you need.

- **Moving highlighted text**   When you need to move something from one part of a document to another, you *could* do it by making a copy, pasting it, and then going back to delete the original. If you do this, however, your colleagues will certainly make fun of you—because there's an easier way. After you highlight what you want to move, select the **Edit**, **Cut** command (the shortcuts are pressing **Ctrl+X** or clicking the **Cut** toolbar button). Your selection disappears from the screen, but don't panic—Windows saves it for you. Position the cursor where you want to place the text, then select **Edit**, **Paste**. Your text miraculously reappears in the new location.

- **Deleting text**   Because even the best typists make occasional typos, knowing how to delete is a necessary editing skill. Put away the correction fluid, though, because deleting a character or two is easier (and less messy) if you use either of the following techniques: Position the cursor to the right of the offending character and press the **Backspace** key, or position the cursor to the left of the character and press the **Delete** key. If you have a large chunk of material you want to expunge from the document, highlight it and press the **Delete** or **Backspace** key.

> **By the Way**
>
> All this cut, copy, and paste moonshine is a bit mysterious. Where does cut text (or whatever) go? How does Windows know what to paste? Does Windows have some kind of digital hip pocket that it uses to store and retrieve cut or copied data? Truth be told, that's not a bad analogy. This "hip pocket" is actually a chunk of your computer's memory called the *clipboard*. When you run the Cut or Copy command, Windows heads to the clipboard, removes whatever currently resides there, and stores the cut or copied data. When you issue the Paste command, Windows grabs whatever is on the clipboard and pastes it into your document.

- **To err is human, to undo divine** What do you do if you paste text to the wrong spot or consign a vital piece of an irreplaceable document to deletion purgatory? Happily, Notepad, WordPad, and many other Windows programs have an Undo feature to get you out of these jams. To reverse your most recent action, select the **Edit**, **Undo** command to restore everything to the way it was before you made your blunder. And yes, there are shortcuts you can use: try either pressing **Ctrl+Z** or clicking the **Undo** toolbar button.

  It's important to remember that most of the time the Undo command usually only undoes your most recent action. So if you delete something, perform some other task, and then try to undo the deletion, chances are the program won't let you do it. Therefore, always try to run **Undo** immediately after making your error. Note, however, that some programs are more flexible and will let you undo several actions. In this case, you just keep selecting the **Undo** command until your document is back the way you want it.

Saving Your Work

"Save your work as soon as you can and as often as you can."

Without even a jot of hyperbole, I'm telling you right here and now that this deceptively simple slogan is probably the single most important piece of advice that you'll stumble upon in this book.

Why all the fuss? When you work with a new or existing document, all the changes you make are stored temporarily in your computer's memory. The bad news is that memory is a fickle and transient medium that, despite its name, forgets all its contents when you turn off the computer. If you haven't saved your document to your hard disk (which maintains its contents even when your computer is turned off), you lose all the changes you've made and it's impossible to get them back. Scary!

To guard against such a disaster, remember my "saving slogan" and keep the following in mind:

- When you create a new document, save it as soon as you've entered any data that's worth keeping.

- After the new document is saved, keep saving it as often as you can. When I'm writing a book, I typically save my work every 30 to 60 seconds (I'm paranoid!), but a reasonable schedule is to save your work every 5 minutes or so.

What Can Go Wrong?

If your computer's memory doesn't go into clean-slate mode until you shut the machine down, you may be wondering why you can't just wait to save until you're ready to close shop for the night. If a power failure shuts off your system or if Windows crashes (these things happen, believe me!), all your unsaved work is toast. By saving constantly, you greatly lessen the chance of that happening.

Saving a New Document

Saving a new document takes a bit of extra work, but after that's out of the way, subsequent saves require only a mouse click or two. To save a new document, follow these steps:

1. Pull down the **File** menu. If you're using WordPad, click the WordPad button (pointed out earlier in Figure 4.1); if you're using Paint, click the **Paint** button, pointed out in Figure 4.2.

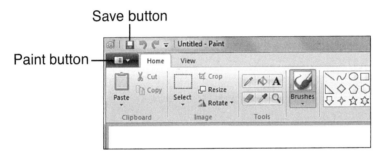

Figure 4.2: In Paint, click the **Paint** button to see the Save command.

2. Click the **Save** command. Alternatively, click the **Save** button in the program's toolbar (see Figure 4.2). The program displays a Save As dialog box like the one shown in Figure 4.3.

3. Use the **File name** text box to enter a name for your document. Note that the name you choose must be different from any other document in the folder. Also, Windows lets you enter filenames that are up to 255 characters long. Your names can include spaces, commas, and apostrophes but not the following characters: \ | ? : * " < > .

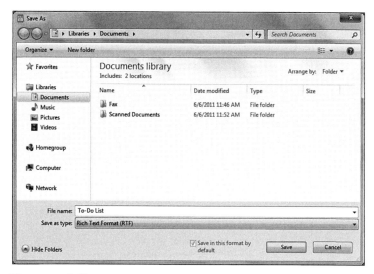

Figure 4.3: The Save As dialog box appears when you're saving a new document.

4. Click the **Save** button. The program makes a permanent copy of the document on your hard disk.

Saving an Existing Document

After all that hard work saving a new document, you'll be happy to know that subsequent saving is much easier. That's because when you select the **File**, **Save** command, the program simply updates the existing hard-disk copy of the document. This takes just a second or two (usually), and no dialog box shows up to pester you for information. Because this is so easy, there's no excuse not to save your work regularly. If you're a fan of keyboard shortcuts, here's one to memorize for the ages: press **Ctrl+S** to save your document. If you're a fan of toolbar buttons, click the **Save** toolbar button instead.

Organizing Your Documents

When you first open the Save As dialog box, the current folder is almost always one of the folders that Windows 7 refers to as a *library*. For example, in Figure 4.3's Save As dialog box, the current folder is the Documents library—which, as you may figure, is a good place to store documents. Windows 7 comes with three other libraries—Music, Pictures, and Videos—and you can pretty much guess what types of files go into each.

I highly recommend that you store all the stuff you create in one of these libraries, because they're designed to be a central storage area for all the files you create. Using libraries is a good idea for three reasons:

- It makes your documents easy to find because you know exactly where they are.

- When you want to back up your documents, you need to only select the libraries (rather than hunting around your hard disk for all your documents).

- Most of the libraries are easy to get to: select **Start** and then click an icon for a specific library: Documents, Pictures, or Music.

These libraries are handy places to store your documents, music, pictures, and videos. However, just as a real library would be in a sorry state of chaos if the librarian just stored the books willy-nilly, so too would each of your computer libraries if you simply saved, say, all your documents harum-scarum in the Documents library.

Just as a brick-and-mortar library divides its books into comprehensible sections (gardening, history, sports, and so on), so you need to divide each of your Windows libraries into sections—technically, they're called *folders*—that you use as storage areas for related documents.

For example, you could start with the Documents library and then create a Letters folder to store your correspondence. You could also create a Lists folder for things such as birthday ideas and Christmas lists, a Notes folder for your jottings, a Shocked and Appalled subfolder to hold your tirades to the newspaper editor, and so on.

The next section takes you through the steps for creating a new folder.

Creating a Folder

There's no time like the present, so let's get right to the steps you need to follow to create a new folder:

1. Open the library in which you want to create your new folder. For example, if you want to put your new folder in Documents, open the Documents library.

2. Click **New Folder** in the taskbar. Windows displays a new subfolder on the screen and displays **New folder** in a text box, as shown in Figure 4.4.

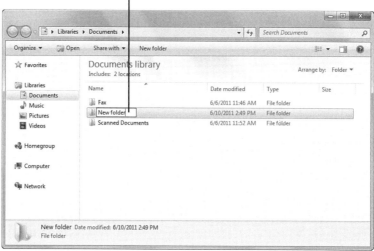

Figure 4.4: When you create a new folder, Windows provides you with a text box so you can enter a proper name for the folder.

3. Because "New folder" isn't a particularly descriptive name, use the text box to type a new name and then press **Enter**. Folder names follow the same rules as filenames: 255 characters maximum, and spaces are okay but the following characters are not: \ | ? : * " < >.

Creating a Copy of a Document

As you work in Windows, you may find that you need to create a second, slightly different copy of a document. For example, you may create a letter and then decide that you need a second copy to send to someone else. Rather than recreating the entire letter from scratch, it's much easier to make a copy of the existing document and then change just the address and salutation.

The easiest way to go about this is to use the Save As command. This command is a lot like Save except that it enables you to save the document with a new name or to a new location. (Think of it as the don't-reinvent-the-wheel command.) To use Save As to create a new document, follow these steps:

1. Open the original document (not a new one). (If you're not sure how to go about this, skip ahead to the section titled, "Opening an Existing Document.")

2. Select the **File**, **Save As** command. The program displays the same Save As dialog box shown earlier in Figure 4.3.

3. Either select a different storage location for the new document or enter a different filename (or both).

4. Click **Save**. The program closes the original document, makes a copy, and then opens the new document.

5. Make your changes to the new document.

Closing a Document

Some weakling Windows programs (such as WordPad and Paint) allow you to open only one document at a time. In such programs, you can close the document you're currently working on by starting a new document, by opening another document, or by quitting the program altogether.

However, most full-featured Windows programs let you open as many documents as you want (subject to the usual memory limitations that govern all computer work). In this case, each open document appears inside its own window—called a *document window*, not surprisingly. These document windows have their own versions of the Minimize, Maximize, Restore, and Close buttons. Also, the name of each document appears on the program's Window menu, which you can use to switch from one document to another.

Because your screen can get crowded pretty fast, though, you probably want to close any documents you don't need at the moment. To do this, activate the document you want to close and select the **File**, **Close** command or click the document window's **Close** button. If you made changes to the document since last saving it, a dialog box appears asking whether you want to save those changes. Click **Yes** to save your changes, **No** to discard the changes, or **Cancel** if you decide to leave the document open.

Opening an Existing Document

After you've saved a document or two, you often need to get one of them back onto the screen to make changes or review your handiwork. To do that, you need to *open* the document by using any of the following techniques.

- **Use the Open dialog box** Select the program's **File, Open** command. (Alternatively, press **Ctrl+O** or click the **Open** toolbar button.) Find the document you want to open, highlight it, and click **Open**.

- **Use a library** If you're using a Windows 7 library to store your stuff, you can open a document by displaying the folder (select **Start** and then click your username), opening the appropriate library (such as Documents or Pictures), and then double-clicking the document's icon. If the appropriate application isn't running, Windows 7 will start it for you and load the document automatically.

- **Use the Search box** Select **Start** and then start typing the name of the document in the Search box. When the name of the document shows up in the search results, click the document to open it.

Locating Documents on Your Computer

Today's computer hard drives come with lots of space, so you can create and store as many documents as you need. That's the good news. The bad news is that the more documents you create and store on your hard drive, the harder it is to find what you need when you need it.

By far, the easiest solution to this file-needle-in-a-hard-drive-haystack conundrum is to use the Start menu's Search box that I mentioned briefly in the previous section. When you type something into the Search box, Windows immediately begins scouring your computer for matching documents. (It also looks for programs, Windows features, contacts, email messages, and more. It's awfully powerful for a simple text box.) And by "matching" documents, I mean any document where the text you've typed appears in the document name or the document text.

For example, suppose you have a file called "Christmas Ideas for Karen" but can't remember where you saved it. That's okay—Windows *does* remember. Click **Start** and then start typing some text that you think will uniquely identify the document (remembering that Windows will look through the document names and the document text). In this case, you might type **karen** into the Search box. Windows then immediately displays any matching documents, as shown in Figure 4.5. From here, you click the one you want, and it opens just like that.

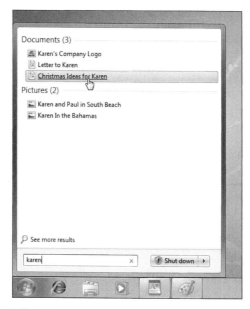

Figure 4.5: When you type some text in the Start menu's Search box, Windows displays a list of the documents that match your typing.

The Least You Need to Know

- To forge a new document, select the **File**, **New** command, press **Ctrl+N**, or click the toolbar's **New** button.
- To save a document, select the **File**, **Save** command, press **Ctrl+S**, or click the toolbar's **Save** button. If you're saving a new document, use the Save As dialog box to pick a location and name for the document.
- You'll simplify your life immeasurably if you store all your files in the libraries provided by Windows 7.
- Press **Backspace** to delete the character to the left of the cursor, press **Delete** to wipe out the character to the right, or press **Ctrl+Z** to undo your most recent mistake.
- To open a document, select the **File**, **Open** command, press **Ctrl+O**, or click the toolbar's **Open** button.
- To locate a document on your computer, click **Start**, type some text that's part of the document name or contents, and then click the document in the search results.

Playing with Photos, Music, and Movies

Chapter 5

In This Chapter

- Transferring photos to your computer
- Understanding photo file formats
- Viewing individual photos and photo slide shows
- Straightening, cropping, and other quick photo fixes
- Burning photos to a CD or DVD
- Playing audio CDs, copying music from a CD, and watching movies

One of the best things about a computer is that it can be a flexible beast when it has to be. That is, although computers are pretty good at letting you read text on the screen and type in your own text creations, modern computers are happy to go way beyond these humble beginnings. Specifically, today's computers excel at what's sometimes called *multimedia*, which is just a fancy-pants way of referring to photos, music, and movies. As you'll see in this chapter, your computer is positively brimming with tools that enable you to copy, view, and even fix photos.

Getting Photos onto Your Computer

It stands to reason that you can't work with photos on your computer if you don't have any photos to work with! Fortunately, however, getting photos into digital form is easier than ever, thanks to three graphics gadgets that have become more affordable:

- A *digital camera* acts much like a regular camera in that it captures and stores a photo of the outside world. The difference is that the digital camera stores the photo internally in its memory instead of on exposed film. It's then possible to connect the digital camera to your computer and save the photo as a graphics file on your hard disk.
- A *scanner* acts much like a photocopier in that it creates an image of a flat surface, such as a photograph or a sheet of paper. The difference is that the scanner saves the image to a graphics file on your hard disk instead of on paper.
- A *memory card* is a small, thin, rectangular wafer designed to store files (particularly photos).

The entire point of a digital camera, scanner, or memory card is to transfer an image of something from the device to your computer's hard drive. From there, you can edit the photo, email it to a friend or colleague, or simply store it for safekeeping. The next three sections show you how to use each device to get photos onto your computer.

Transfer Photos from a Digital Camera

Although it's occasionally fun to browse photos on your digital camera, the photos are too tiny to be satisfying. If you want to take a good peek at your handiwork, you need to get those pics onto your computer.

Fortunately, Windows gives you not one but *two* ways to go about this: you can use Windows itself, or you can use Windows Live Photo Gallery.

To use Windows, follow these easier-done-than-said steps:

1. Connect your digital camera to your computer. (You learned how to do this back in Chapter 1.) After a few seconds, the AutoPlay dialog box appears, as shown in Figure 5.1.

By the Way

If for some reason you don't see the AutoPlay dialog box, select **Start**, **Computer** to open the Computer window, where you'll see an icon for your camera. Right-click the camera icon, click **Import pictures and videos**, and skip to step 3.

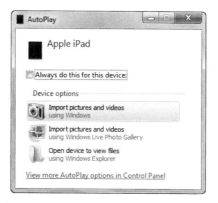

Figure 5.1: The AutoPlay dialog box appears a few seconds after you connect your digital camera.

2. Click **Import pictures and videos using Windows**. Windows offers the Import Pictures and Videos dialog box, shown in Figure 5.2.

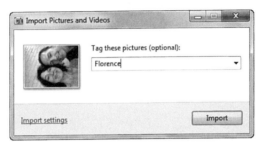

Figure 5.2: Use this dialog box to get your Windows digital camera import underway.

3. Use the **Tag these pictures** text box to type a word or short phrase that describes the pictures. This is called a *tag*, and Windows uses the tag as follows:

   - It creates a subfolder in the My Pictures folder, and the name of the new subfolder is today's date followed by your tag. For example, if today is August 23, 2012, and your tag is "Florence," then the new subfolder will have the following name: 2012-08-23 Florence.
   - It gives the file the same name as the tag, with the number 001 after it, like so: Florence 001.jpg.

   If you're importing a bunch of photos from your digital camera, then the number gets bumped up for each photo: 002, 003, and so on.

4. Click **Import**. Windows starts moving the photos from the camera to your PC. If you want Windows to delete the photos from the camera when it's done, activate the **Erase after importing** check box. When the import is complete, Windows drops you off in the Imported Pictures and Videos folder.

If you've downloaded Windows Live Photo Gallery from the Windows Live Essentials website (as I talked about back in Chapter 3), you can use that program to handle your importing chores. Here's how it works:

1. Connect your digital camera to your computer. After a few seconds, the AutoPlay dialog box appears.

2. Click **Import pictures and videos using Windows Live Photo Gallery**. Windows offers the Import Pictures and Videos dialog box, shown in Figure 5.2.

> **By the Way**
>
> If the AutoPlay dialog box doesn't appear, select **Start**, **All Programs**, **Windows Live Photo Gallery** to get the program up and running, click the **Home** tab, click **Import**, and continue with step 3.

3. Click the icon for your digital camera, then click **Import**. The Import Photos and Videos dialog box shown in Figure 5.3 appears.

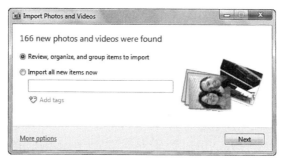

Figure 5.3: Use this dialog box to perform your Windows Live Photo Gallery importing duties.

4. Click the **Import all new items now** option.

5. Type a name for the import in the text box. (This will be the name of the folder that Windows Live Photo Gallery creates to store the imported photos.)

6. Click **Import**. Windows Live Photo Gallery starts importing the photos from the camera to your computer. If you want Windows Live Photo Gallery to delete the photos from the camera when the dust clears, activate the **Erase after importing** check box. When the import is complete, Windows drops you off in the Imported Pictures and Videos folder.

Scan a Photo

Windows comes with its own Scanner and Camera Wizard to give you a step-by-step method for capturing photos. Let's see how it works. First, place the photo face-down on the scanner glass. Then, launch the Scanner and Camera Wizard using one of the following methods:

- Your device should have some kind of "scan" button, so press that button.

- Select **Start**, **Devices and Printers**, click your scanner, and then click **Start scan**.

- In Windows Live Photo Gallery (select **Start**, **All Programs**, **Windows Live Photo Gallery**), click the **Home** tab, then click **Import**. In the Import Pictures and Videos dialog box, click your scanner and then click **Import**.

- Select **Start**, **All Programs**, **Windows Fax and Scan**. In the Windows Fax and Scan window, select **File**, **New**, **Scan**, click your scanner, and then click **OK**.

Whichever method you choose, you see the New Scan dialog box. Feel free to click the **Preview** button to make sure your photo is straight.

After the preview appears, chances are you'll see lots of white space around the photo and a dashed line around the border of that white space. This dashed border defines the area that will be scanned. You don't want to include the white space with your scanned photo, so use your mouse to click and drag the corners of the dashed border so that it surrounds only the photo, as shown in Figure 5.4.

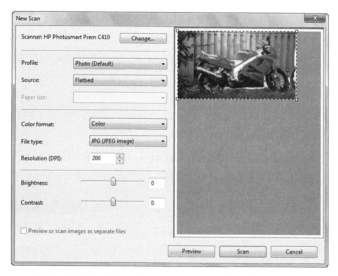

Figure 5.4: Click **Preview** to get a look at your photo, then click and drag the dashed border so that it surrounds only your photo.

When you're ready, click **Scan**. After Windows scans the photo, the Import Pictures and Videos dialog box appears. Type a tag for the photo, then click **Import**.

Transfer Photos from a Memory Card

Many digital cameras store photos using a memory card. These miniature memory modules come in many different shapes and sizes, and they come with names such as CompactFlash, MultiMedia, Memory Stick, or SecureDigital. They're handy little devils because after you transfer your photos to your computer, you can delete the photos from the card and start all over again. Although you usually get at the card's photos by connecting the camera directly to your computer (as described earlier), you can also insert a memory card into a memory card reader and then transfer the card's contents to the computer. Most new computers come with a built-in memory card reader, which appears as a collection of narrow slots on the front of the computer. If your computer doesn't have a built-in reader, you can purchase a separate reader and then connect it—usually to a USB port.

Each slot in the memory card reader is designed to handle a particular type of card. Helpfully, most cards will only fit into a particular slot, so you just need to find the one that fits whatever memory card you have.

Windows treats each slot in a memory card reader as a disk drive, and they show up in the Computer folder as Removable Disk drives. You're then free to insert a memory card and browse its photos directly, as described in the next section. In some cases, however, inserting the memory card prompts Windows to display the dialog box shown in Figure 5.5.

Windows wants to know just what the heck you'd like to do with the photos on the card, so click the action you prefer. If you want to make this the default action, activate the **Always do this for pictures** check box.

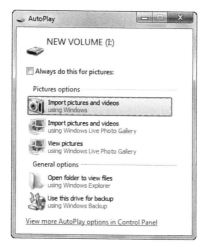

Figure 5.5: When you insert a memory card, Windows may display this dialog box.

In particular, if you want to copy the card's photos to your hard disk, follow these steps:

1. Click the **Import pictures and videos using Windows** command. The Import Pictures and Videos dialog box appears.

2. To apply a tag to all photos, type the tag in the **Tag these pictures** text box.

3. Click **Import**. Windows begins importing the photos.

4. If you also want Windows to remove the photos from the memory card when the import is complete, activate the **Erase after importing** check box.

By the Way

If you have Windows Live Photo Gallery installed, an alternative method is to click **Import pictures and videos using Windows Live Photo Gallery** in the AutoPlay dialog box. Click the **Import all new items now** option, type a name for the import in the text box, and click **Import**.

Photo File Formats

Few things get the man (or woman) on the street more thoroughly bamboozled than the bewildering array of file formats (also known as file types) that exist in the digital world. And perhaps the worst culprit is the photo file category, which boasts an unseemly large number of formats. My goal in this section is to help you get through the thicket of acronyms and minutiae that characterize photo file formats and show you how to simplify things.

Before you go any further into this file-format business, you may enjoy taking a step or two in reverse to consider the bigger picture: What is a file format, and why do we need so many of them? I like to look at file formats as the underlying structure of a file that's akin to a car's underlying structure. The latter is a collection of metal and plastic bits that form the frame, axles, suspension, engine, and other innards that determine how the car performs. A file format is similar in that it consists of a collection of bits and bytes that determines how the photo is viewed. As you'll see, some formats are better suited for displaying photos while others are better suited to line drawings.

The sigh-of-relief-inducing news is that although the computing world is on speaking terms with dozens of different photo formats, Windows is conversant with only five:

- **Bitmap.** This is the standard photo file format used by Windows. It's good for color drawings, although its files tend to be on the large side. Bitmap photo files use the .bmp extension, so these files are also referred to sometimes as BMP files.

- **GIF.** This is one of the standard graphics file formats used on the internet. It's only capable of storing 256 colors, so it's suitable for relatively simple line drawings or for photos that use only a few colors. The resulting files are compressed, so they end up quite a bit smaller than bitmap files.

- **JPEG (or JPG).** This is the other standard graphics file format that you see on the World Wide Web. This format can reproduce millions of colors, so it's suitable for photographs and other high-quality images. JPEG (it's pronounced JAY-peg) stores photos in a compressed format, so it can knock high-quality photos down to a manageable size while still retaining some picture fidelity. (However, the more you compress the photo, the poorer the photo quality becomes.)

- **PNG.** This is a relatively new file format that's becoming more popular on the internet. It's a versatile format that can be used with both simple drawings and photos. For the latter, PNG supports compression to keep photos relatively small. (And, unlike JPEG, the PNG compression doesn't reduce the quality of the photo.)

- **TIF.** This format is often used with photo scanners and digital cameras because it does a great job of rendering photos and other scanned photos. The downside is that this format doesn't usually compress the photos in any way, so it creates *huge* files. (Note that this file format sometimes goes by the name of TIFF instead of just TIF.)

So which one should you use when creating your own photo files? That depends:

- If you're scanning a photo or downloading a photo from a digital camera for printing or for editing only on your computer, use TIF or JPEG.

- If you're scanning a photo or downloading a photo from a digital camera for emailing or publishing on the internet, use JPEG.

- If you're creating a drawing that you'll print out or work with only on your computer, use the bitmap format.

- If you're creating a simple drawing that you'll be publishing on the World Wide Web, use GIF.

- If you're creating a more complex drawing that you'll be publishing to the internet, use PNG.

Viewing Photos

Back in Chapter 3, I told you about your main user account folder and mentioned that it's the perfect spot to store the documents you create. If you've been doing that, then you no doubt have noticed that your user folder includes a library named Pictures—and you probably guessed that this subfolder is where you should be hoarding your picture files. That's certainly true, but not just because of the library's name. Pictures is the place to squirrel away your photos because it's a special library that "understands" picture files—and therefore offers you some extra features that are designed specifically for messing around with photos:

- Offers "thumbnail" versions of each photo that show you not only the name of each file but also give you a miniature preview of what each photo looks like

- Enables you to see a "preview" of any photo, from which you can then rotate the photo, print it, and perform a few other tasks

- Enables you to view all your photos one by one in a kind of "slide show"

- Enables you to set up a particular photo as your Windows desktop background

Most of the rest of this chapter takes you through the specifics of these features. Before getting to that, however, it's probably a good idea to review how you get to the Pictures library. Windows offers two methods:

- Select **Start**, **Pictures**.
- If you're currently in your main user folder (Libraries), double-click the icon for the **Pictures** library.

By the Way

If you're using an earlier version of Windows, remember that these versions don't use libraries—they just use regular folders. Also, if you're using Windows XP, you get to your pictures by selecting **Start**, **My Pictures**.

Looking Through Your Photos

When you arrive at the Pictures folder, you'll probably see icons for various subfolders. If so, double-click the subfolder you want to view.

You'll now see the photo files arranged something like those shown in Figure 5.6. That is, instead of a boring (and only marginally useful) icon, each file shows a mini-preview of the photo contained in the file.

In this handy way of looking at things, the little preview of each photo is called a *thumbnail*, and Windows displays photo thumbnails no matter which view you use (even Details).

Definition

A **thumbnail** is a scaled-down preview of a photo or other type of file.

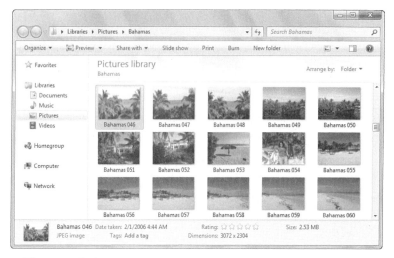

Figure 5.6: By default, Windows displays a small preview of each graphics file in the Pictures folder.

If you want to know details about a photo—such as its height and width in pixels, its file type, and its size—click the file. The details then appear in the Preview pane at the bottom of the window (see Figure 5.6).

You should also note at this point that when you click a photo file to select it, the folder window displays several photo-related links, including **Preview** and **Slide show**. I'll talk about these links as you work through this chapter.

If you prefer to work with one photo at a time, the photo preview feature might be just what you're looking for. To activate it, select the photo you want to work with and then click **Preview** (an alternative method is to double-click the photo). This loads the picture into the Windows Photo Viewer window, shown in Figure 5.7.

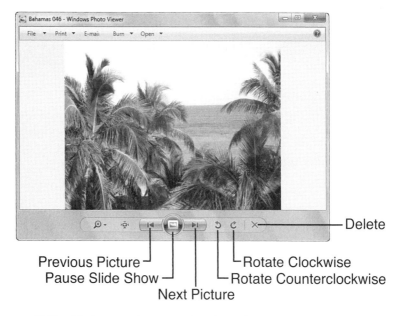

Figure 5.7: Click **Preview** to display the selected file in the Photo Viewer.

This window shows you a larger version of the photo and is also festooned with a few icons at the bottom:

- **Previous.** Click this icon to display the previous photo in the Pictures folder.

- **Play Slide Show.** Click this icon (or press **F11**) to start a slide show of the files in the Pictures folder (more on this later in the chapter).

- **Next Picture.** Click this icon to display the next photo in the Pictures folder.

- **Rotate Clockwise.** Click this icon to rotate the photo clockwise 90 degrees. Note that this rotation doesn't apply only to the preview; Windows applies it to the file itself.

- **Rotate Counterclockwise.** Click this icon to rotate the photo counterclockwise 90 degrees. Again, this change is applied to the file itself.

- **Delete.** Click this icon (or press **Delete**) to send the photo to the Recycle Bin.

> **By the Way**
>
> You can also jump to the previous picture by pressing the **left-arrow key** on your keyboard. For the next picture, press the **right-arrow key**. Note, too, that you can also rotate the photo counterclockwise by pressing **Ctrl+,** (comma) and you can rotate the photo clockwise by pressing **Ctrl+.** (period).

Watching a Photo Slide Show

For its next trick, the Pictures library also offers a "slide show" view. This means that Windows displays a full-screen version of the first file, waits a few seconds, displays the second file, and so on. To activate the slide show, you have two choices:

- In the Pictures folder, click the **Slide show** link.
- In the Windows Photo Viewer window, click the **Play Slide Show** icon.

Note that you can also control the slide show by hand by right-clicking the screen to display the following commands:

- **Play.** Restarts a paused slide show.
- **Pause.** Pauses the slide show.

- **Next.** Displays the next photo (you can also press **right arrow**).
- **Back.** Displays the previous photo (you can also press **left arrow**).
- **Shuffle.** Shows the pictures in random order.
- **Loop.** Starts over from the beginning when it has run through all the pictures.
- **Slide Show Speed.** These commands control the playback speed: Slow, Medium, or Fast.
- **Exit.** Stops the slide show (you can also press **Esc**).

Fixing Your Photos

Windows Live Photo Gallery comes with a limited set of tools for altering photos. Select **Start**, **All Programs**, **Windows Live Photo Gallery** to start the program, double-click the photo you want to work with, and then click the **Edit** tab. As you can see in Figure 5.8, there are a bunch of tools available here, but the next three sections cover the most popular choices: straightening a photo, removing red eye, and cropping a photo.

Good to Know!

If, like me, you really don't know what the heck you're doing when it comes to things like "color temperature" and exposure, you can also click **Auto adjust** to have Windows Live Photo Gallery make the adjustments for you.

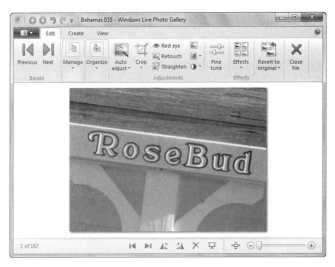

Figure 5.8: Double-click a photo to open it and see the Windows Live Photo Gallery's tools for fixing photos.

Straighten a Photo

Few of us use a tripod when taking pictures, so unless you have a steady hand, getting your camera perfectly level when you take a shot can be quite hard. This means that, for most of us, at least a few of our photos will turn out a bit (or sometimes a lot) crooked. To fix this problem, you can use Windows Live Photo Gallery to automatically rotate the photo just enough to make everything appear level.

Open Windows Live Photo Gallery and double-click your photo to open it. Click the **Edit** tab, then click **Straighten**. Figure 5.9 shows the same photo from Figure 5.8 after I clicked the Straighten button.

Chapter 5: Playing with Photos, Music, and Movies **101**

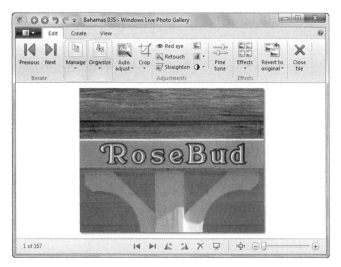

Figure 5.9: After using the Straighten tool, the photo from Figure 5.8 is now picture-perfect.

Remove Red Eye

In situations where you don't have lots of light, your camera will automatically use its built-in flash to generate some artificial light and ensure that you can see the people you're photographing. That's a good thing, but the flash often has an annoying tendency to reflect off the subjects' retinas. The result is the common (and not particularly attractive) phenomenon of red eye, where each person's pupils appear as red instead of black.

Here's how you get rid of red eye:

1. Open Windows Live Photo Gallery and double-click your photo to open it.
2. Click the **View** tab.

3. Click **Zoom In** a few times to magnify the image and get a good look at the red eye you want to remove. Note that you may have to use your mouse to click and drag the photo to bring the red eye into view.

4. Click the **Edit** tab.

5. Click **Red eye**.

6. Use your mouse to click and drag a small rectangle around one of the red-eye examples. Ideally, your rectangle should be just large enough to enclose the pupil. When you release the mouse, Windows Live Photo Gallery removes the red eye. Figure 5.10 shows a photo where the eye on the right has had the red eye removed and the eye on the left has the red-eye rectangle around its pupil.

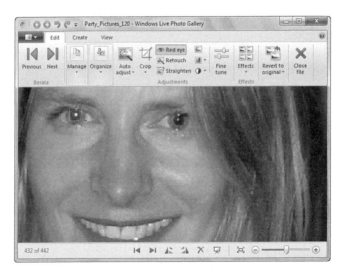

Figure 5.10: Click the Red eye tool and then click and drag a rectangle around each red pupil.

Crop Out Unwanted Elements

We've all taken photos that end up with extraneous elements at the edges. It may be an overhead wire you didn't notice, a person's hand or head inadvertently sneaking into your frame, or—all too commonly for some of us—our own thumb.

Fortunately, your photo isn't necessarily marred for life, because you can often cut out those extra elements—a process called *cropping*. When you crop a photo, you specify a rectangular area of the photo that you want to keep. Windows Live Photo Gallery discards everything outside the rectangle.

Follow these steps to crop out unwanted elements from a photo:

1. Open Windows Live Photo Gallery and double-click your photo to open it.

2. Click the **Edit** tab.

3. Click the top half of the **Crop** button. Windows Live Photo Gallery displays a grid on your photo.

4. Adjust the position and size of the grid so that it covers just the portion of your photo that you want to keep:

    - To move the grid, place the mouse pointer anywhere inside the grid (it changes to a four-headed arrow), then click and drag to move the grid into position.

    - To size the grid, position the mouse pointer over any of the small squares that you see on the edges of the grid, then click and drag the square to adjust the edges to the size you want.

5. Click the lower half of the **Crop** button, then click **Apply crop**.

> **Good to Know!**
>
> It's often the case that you have a particular photo size in mind, such as 5 × 7 or 8 × 10. In such cases, you can set the cropping grid to the size you want, then move it into the best position. To set a specific cropping grid size, click the lower half of the **Crop** button, click **Proportion**, and then click the size you want.

Figure 5.11 shows a photo with an extraneous element on the right and a grid set up to crop out that element.

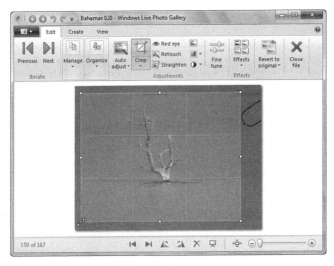

Figure 5.11: Click the **Crop** button, then adjust the position and size of the grid to define the area you want to keep.

Copying Photos to a CD or DVD

You can copy a selection of photos to a recordable CD or DVD disc—a process called *burning*. You can then send the disc to a friend or relative to share your photos.

If you have a CD or DVD burner—that is, a CD or DVD drive capable of recording data to a disc—attached to your computer (almost all new computers come with one), Windows should recognize it and be ready to burn at will. To try this, you first have to set up the disc by following these steps:

1. Insert a blank CD into your CD burner (or a blank CD or DVD into your DVD burner). (If the AutoPlay window shows up, click **Close** to get rid of it.)

2. Select **Start, Computer** and then double-click the CD or DVD drive. The first time you do this, the Burn a Disc dialog box appears.

3. Type a disc title, make sure the **Like a USB flash drive** option is selected, and click **Next**. Windows formats the disc to make it ready to receive files. This may take a while, so groom your dog while you wait.

When all that malarkey is done (again, if you're pestered by the AutoPlay window, just click **Close**), you're ready to get down to the burning thing by following these steps:

1. In Windows Explorer, open a folder that contains one or more of the photos you want to burn.

2. Select the photos you want to burn to the disc.

3. Click **Burn** in the taskbar. Windows copies the files to the disc.

4. Repeat steps 1 to 3 until you've sent all the files you want to the disc.

5. Select **Start, Computer** and then double-click the disc to open it.

6. Click **Close session**. Windows finalizes the disc burning.

7. Click **Eject**. Windows spits out the disc.

Working with Other Types of Media

The graphics you learned about in the first part of this chapter represent only a selection of Windows's media treats. There are actually quite a few more goodies that fall into the "sights for sore eyes" category—and even a few that could be called "sounds for sore ears." In the rest of this chapter, you see how Windows can turn your lowly computer into a multimedia powerhouse capable of playing audio CDs, copying music from a CD, and watching movies.

Listening to an Audio CD

If you like to listen to music while you use your computer, it's possible to convince Media Player to crank up an audio CD. Audio CDs use the same dimensions as CD-ROMs, so any audio CD will fit snugly inside your CD or DVD drive (if you have one). From there, you use the Media Player application to play the CD's tracks.

When you insert your audio CD, you see the Now Playing window a few seconds later, and the CD starts playing automatically. To control the playback, move the mouse pointer over the Now Playing window to display the controls, as shown in Figure 5.12 (which also points out the name of each control).

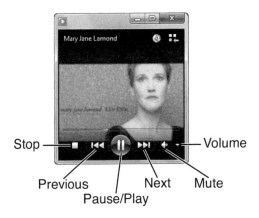

Figure 5.12: Move the mouse pointer over the Now Playing window to see the playback controls.

Use the following to control the playback of the audio CD:

- **Stop.** Stops the playback.
- **Previous.** Skips back to the previous song on the CD.
- **Pause/Play.** Pauses and resumes the playback.
- **Next.** Skips ahead to the next song on the CD.
- **Mute.** Turns off the playback volume. Click this button again to restore the volume.
- **Volume.** Sets the playback volume. Click this button to display the volume slider, then click and drag the little blue ball to set the volume level.

When you're done with the CD, select **Start**, **Computer**, right-click the CD, and then click **Eject**.

Copying Music from an Audio CD

Media Player's audio CD playback is flexible, for sure, but audio-CD playback suffers from two important drawbacks:

- Shuffling discs in and out of the drive can be a hassle.
- There isn't any way to mix tunes from two or more CDs, even in the unlikely event that your system has multiple CD and/or DVD drives.

To solve these dilemmas, Media Player enables you to copy—or *rip*, as the kids say—individual tracks from one or more CDs and store them on your computer's hard disk. From there, you can listen to your music directly from your computer whenever you feel like it.

To perform the rip, insert the audio CD, wait until you see the Now Playing window, move your mouse over the window to display the controls, then click **Rip CD** (pointed out in Figure 5.13).

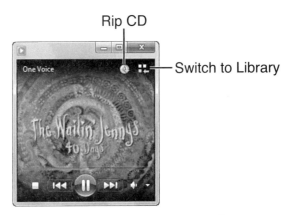

Figure 5.13: Move the mouse pointer over the Now Playing window, then click **Rip CD**.

If you want to watch the progress of the rip, move the mouse pointer over the Now Playing window and then click **Switch to Library** (shown in Figure 5.13). This displays the full Windows Media Player window. As you can see in Figure 5.14, the Rip status column tells you when each track has been "Ripped to library."

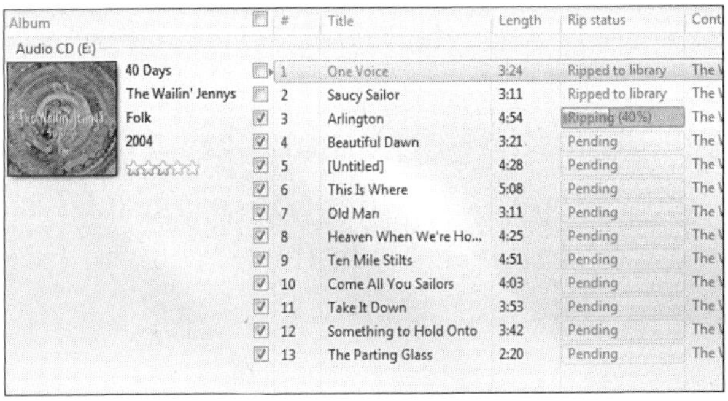

Figure 5.14: In Windows Media Player, the Rip status column tells when each track has been ripped to your computer.

Watching DVD Movies

You may be surprised to hear that you can watch full-length feature films right on your computer! Once again, the Windows Media Player program does the heavy lifting here, and for the most part all you have to do is sit back and enjoy.

Go ahead and insert the DVD. After a few seconds, Media Player springs into action and automatically starts playing the movie. For the best viewing experience, Media Player uses the entire screen to play the movie. This is called full-screen mode, but you can exit this mode any time you like (as described later in this section).

To control the playback, move the mouse to display the controls pointed out in Figure 5.15.

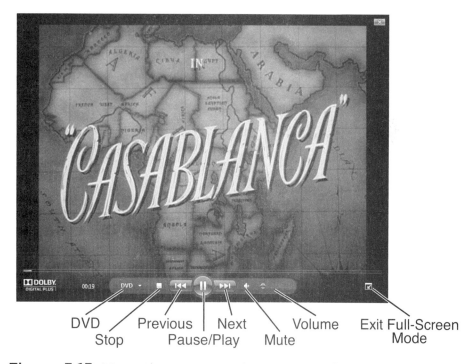

Figure 5.15: Move the mouse pointer to see the movie playback controls.

Here's a summary of the controls you get to use:

- **DVD.** Click this button to access the features of the DVD, such as the main menu and Closed Captioning.
- **Stop.** Stops the movie and returns you to the beginning of the show. You can also press **Ctrl+S**.
- **Previous.** Skips to the previous chapter of the DVD. You can also press **Ctrl+B**.
- **Pause/Play.** Pauses the movie while it's playing; restarts a paused movie. You can also press **Ctrl+P**.
- **Next.** Skips to the next chapter of the DVD. You can also press **Ctrl+F**.

> **Good to Know!**
>
> If you want to fast-forward through the movie, press and hold down the left mouse button over **Next**, or press **Ctrl+Shift+F**. To rewind instead, press and hold down the left mouse button over **Back** or press **Ctrl+Shift+B**.

- **Mute.** Turns off the sound. You can also press **F7**.
- **Volume.** Controls the playback volume. Drag the slider to the left to reduce the volume or to the right to increase the volume. You can also press **F9** to increase the volume or press **F8** to decrease the volume.
- **Exit Full-Screen Mode.** Leaves full-screen mode and displays the movie in a regular window. You can also press **Esc**.

When you're done with the DVD, select **Start**, **Computer**, right-click the DVD, and then click **Eject**.

The Least You Need to Know

- To get pictures from a camera, connect the camera and then use the AutoPlay dialog box to click either **Import pictures and videos using Windows** or **Import pictures and videos using Windows Live Photo Gallery**.
- To scan a photo, either press the device's "scan" button or select **Start**, **Devices and Printers**, click your scanner, and then click **Start scan**.
- If you're working with photos only on your computer or printing them out, the best photo format to use is TIF. If you're going to email photos or publish them on the internet, use the JPEG format.
- In the Pictures folder, click **Preview** to load the selected photo into the Photo Viewer.
- To burn data to a formatted CD or DVD, select the files and folders and then click the **Burn** button in the taskbar.
- To listen to an audio CD or watch a DVD movie, insert the disc and Media Player will start the playback automatically.

Troubleshooting Your Computer

Chapter 6

In This Chapter

- Setting up your system for easier recovery by backing up your files
- Determining the source of a problem
- Troubleshooting problems using websites and newsgroups
- Using general troubleshooting strategies to solve common problems
- Recovering everything from a single file to your entire system

We live in a world where most things work well most of the time. That's a good thing, because having things work well certainly makes your life easier and less stressful—but it's that little word *most* that inevitably interrupts your easy and stress-free life. *Most* means that, occasionally, things do *not* work well—and depending on how much you rely on whatever is causing the problem, much hair pulling and gnashing of teeth can ensue.

I probably don't have to tell you that computers fall well within this works-well-most-of-the-time world. Computers are incredibly complex machines, so it's just this side of miraculous that they can go without a glitch for days—and sometimes even weeks on end.

But this blissful computing experience eventually ends for all of us, and when a problem crops up, you need to get it solved—fast. Some computer problems require professional expertise to set right, but you'd be surprised at how many tools you have at your fingertips to solve some computing woes on your own. This chapter takes you through a few of those tools and also looks at a few specific problems.

Backing Up Your Computer

Before we get to the problems, let's first talk about something you need to do *now* to make it easier to recover from problems down the road. First, here's a story.

A few years ago, I turned on my computer in anticipation of another day's writing fun. I heard a couple alarming beeps and then saw a **Hard disk configuration error** message on my screen. My hard disk had died a horrible death, and there was nothing I could do about it. The worst part was that I had hundreds of documents on the disk that were now gone for good because I'd been too lazy to back up my files. It took me weeks to recover from that disaster, and I've been a rabid backer-upper up ever since.

I found out the hard way that there are two types of computer users: those who back up their documents and those who eventually wish they had. If you learn anything at all from this book, I hope it's this: someday, sometime, somewhere, some sort of evil will befall your computer and all your data will be trashed. So be prepared by using the ever-so-easy Backup tool that comes with Windows 7. Why is it so easy? Because you configure it once, and then subsequent backups happen automatically so you never have to think about it again. This section shows you how it works.

Backup to an External Hard Drive

First, you should know that for the easiest backup experience, you need to add some equipment to your computer. Specifically, you need to attach an external hard drive, which will plug into a USB port on your computer and then be ready to go in seconds flat (see Chapter 1 for more details). The external hard drives they sell these days are big enough to hold all your backup data and are fast enough that each backup won't take forever.

Good to Know!

You don't need to get the biggest external hard drive you can find. For most systems, a 500 GB drive is more than enough.

When you attach the drive, the AutoPlay dialog box appears, as shown in Figure 6.1. This is good, because it tells you the name of the drive and which letter the drive uses. For example, in Figure 6.1 you can see that the drive is named "External HD" and its letter is "E." You'll need this information when you configure your backups. Once you've made a note (mental or otherwise) of the name and letter, click the **Close** button (the **X**) to close the AutoPlay dialog box.

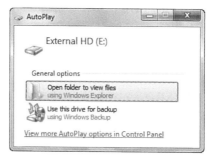

Figure 6.1: After you connect the external hard drive, use the AutoPlay dialog box to make a note of the drive's name and letter.

Configuring the Backup

With that out of the way, let's whip out the brass tacks and get down to business. To get started, select **Start**, **All Programs**, **Maintenance**, **Backup and Restore**. After a second or two, the Backup and Restore window appears—as shown in Figure 6.2.

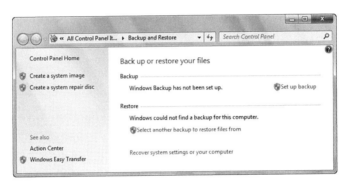

Figure 6.2: Use the Backup and Restore window to configure your backups.

Your first job is to configure the Automatic Backup feature, which requires just a few steps:

1. Click **Set up backup**. The Set Up Backup Wizard pulls itself out of a hat and asks you to choose where you want your document backed up.

2. In the list of drives, click the external drive that you attached (see Figure 6.3), then click **Next** when you're ready to move on. The What do you want to back up? dialog box appears.

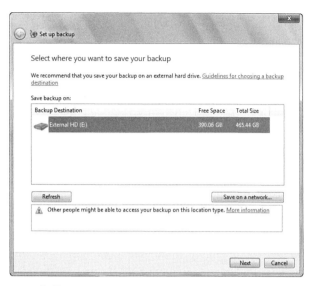

Figure 6.3: In this dialog box, click your external hard drive.

3. Your best (and easiest) bet here is to leave the **Let Windows choose** option selected, then click **Next**. The Review your backup settings dialog box appears.

4. That's about it. Click **Save settings and run backup** to give the wizard its walking papers. Windows Backup gets down to business and backs up your computer.

5. When the backup is done, click **Close**.

You'll need the Backup and Restore window for the next section, so leave it on your desktop for now.

Creating a System Repair Disc

If, as the old saw has it, an ounce of prevention is worth a pound of cure, then configuring Windows 7's automatic backup feature places you squarely in what I like to call ounce-of-prevention mode. While you're in that mode, there's a second bit of preventative maintenance that you can do: create a system repair disc. This is a CD or DVD that you can use in the event that your computer simply refuses to start. In this case, you start the computer using the system repair disc instead, and the disc contains tools that will help you get your computer back on its feet.

Follow these steps to create a system repair disc:

1. If you don't already have the Backup and Restore window onscreen, select **Start**, **All Programs**, **Maintenance**, **Backup and Restore**.

2. Click **Create a system repair disc**.

3. Insert a blank CD or DVD into your computer's CD/DVD drive.

4. Click **Create disc**. Windows copies some files to the disc, which takes a few minutes.

5. When Windows lets you know it has finished creating the disc, click **Close**.

6. Click **OK** to return to the Backup and Restore window.

7. Select **Start**, **Computer**.

8. Right-click your CD/DVD drive, then click **Eject**. Windows ejects your repair disc.

9. Use a permanent marker to write "Repair Disc" or something similar on the disc so you'll remember what it's for. Be sure to save the disc in a safe place.

How to Troubleshoot a Problem

As I've said, computer problems are pretty much inevitable, so you need to know how to troubleshoot and resolve any woes that invariably will come your way. In this section (indeed, in the rest of this chapter), I help you do just that by showing you my favorite techniques for determining problem sources.

Determine the Source of the Problem

One of the ongoing mysteries that all computer users experience at one time or another is what can be called the now-you-see-it-now-you-don't problem. This is a glitch that plagues you for a while and then mysteriously vanishes without any intervention on your part. (This also tends to occur when you ask a nearby user or computer repairperson to look at the problem. Like the automotive problem that goes away when you take the car to a mechanic, computer problems will often resolve themselves as soon as a knowledgeable user sits down at the keyboard.) When this happens, most people just shake their heads and resume working—grateful to no longer have to deal with the problem.

Unfortunately, most computer ills don't get resolved so easily. For these more intractable problems, your first order of business is to track down the source of the snag. This is, at best, a hit-or-miss effort, but it can be done if you take a systematic approach. Over the years, I've found that the best method is to ask a series of questions designed to gather the required information and/or to narrow down clues to the culprit. Here are the questions:

- **Did you get an error message?** Unfortunately, most computer error messages are obscure and do little to help you resolve a problem directly. However, error codes and error text can help you down the road, either by giving you something to search for in an online database (see "Online Resources" later in this chapter) or by providing information to a tech support person. Therefore, you should always write down the full text of any error message that appears.

- **Did you recently change any Windows settings?** If the problem started after you changed your Windows configuration, try reversing the change. Even something as seemingly innocent as starting the screen saver can cause problems, so don't rule anything out.

- **Did you recently change any application settings?** If so, try reversing the change to see whether it solves the problem. If that doesn't help, check to see whether an upgrade is available. Also, some applications come with a "Repair" option that can fix corrupted files. Otherwise, try reinstalling the program.

- **Did you recently install a new program?** If you suspect a new program is causing system instability, restart your computer and try using the system for a while without running the new program. If the problem doesn't reoccur, then the new program is likely the culprit. Try using the program without any other programs running. Again, you can also try the program's "Repair" option, or you can reinstall the program.

- **Did you recently upgrade an existing program?** If so, try uninstalling the upgrade.

- **Did you recently apply an update from Windows Update?** Updates rarely make things worse (thankfully, because they're *supposed* to make things better), but nothing is certain in the Windows world. If your machine has been discombobulated since you installed an update, try removing the update. Select **Start**, **Control Panel**, **Programs**, **View installed updates** to display the Installed Updates window. Select the update that you want to trash, then select **Remove**.

- **Did you recently install a Windows 7 service pack?** If you installed a *service pack* and you elected to save the old system files, then you can uninstall the service pack using Control Panel's Installed Programs window (as described in Chapter 3).

Definition

A **service pack** is a Windows update that includes problem fixes, security enhancements, new features, and other changes designed to make Windows run better.

Try Some General Troubleshooting Tips

Figuring out the cause of a problem is often the hardest part of troubleshooting, but by itself it doesn't do you much good. Once you know the source, you need to parlay that information into a fix for the problem. I discussed a few solutions in the previous section, but here are a few other general fixes you need to keep in mind:

- **Close all programs** You can often fix flaky behavior by shutting down all your open programs and starting again. This is a particularly useful fix for problems caused by low memory or low system resources.

- **Log off Windows** Logging off clears the memory and gives you a slightly cleaner slate than merely closing all your programs.

- **Restart the computer** If problems exist with some system files and devices, logging off won't help because these objects remain loaded. By restarting the system (as I described in Chapter 2), you reload the entire system—which is often enough to solve many computer problems.

- **Turn off the computer and restart** You can often solve a hardware problem by first shutting your machine off. Wait for 30 seconds to give all devices time to spin down, then restart. To shut down Windows, click **Start** and then click **Shut Down**.

- **Check connections, power switches, and so on** Some of the most common (and embarrassing) causes of hardware problems are the simple physical things: making sure a device is turned on, checking that cable connections are secure, and ensuring that insertable devices are properly inserted.

Run Windows's Troubleshooters

Windows 7 comes with a few features called *troubleshooters* that are designed to tackle problems using simple, step-by-step procedures. Select **Start**, **Control Panel**, then click the **Find and fix problems** link under the System and Security heading. The Troubleshooting window offers a bunch of problem-solving tools for topics such as programs, hardware, system, and security. The idea is that you click a topic related to your problem, and the troubleshooter will take you step-by-step through one or more possible solutions.

Let's try an example. One problem that may crop up from time to time is that a program that was designed to run under a previous version of Windows refuses to run under Windows 7. Rather than shell out even more money buying a Windows 7–compatible version of the program, in many cases you can configure the program to work properly under Windows 7. This configuration is made easy by a Windows 7 troubleshooter:

1. In the Troubleshooting window, click **Run programs made for previous versions of Windows**. The Program Compatibility troubleshooter appears.

2. Click **Next**. The Program Compatibility troubleshooter displays a list of programs.

3. Click the program that won't work, then click **Next**. The Program Compatibility troubleshooter asks you to choose a troubleshooting option.

4. Click **Try recommended settings**. The Program Compatibility troubleshooter analyzes the program and then applies a setting that should allow the program to run properly. In Figure 6.4, for example, you can see that the troubleshooter configured the program so that when it runs, it thinks it's actually running under Windows XP.

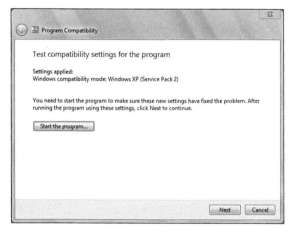

Figure 6.4: Use the Program Compatibility troubleshooter to make a program designed for a previous version of Windows run correctly under Windows 7.

5. Click **Start the program**. If Windows warns you about making changes to the program, click **OK**.

6. Return to the troubleshooter, then click **Next**.

7. If the program starts without a hitch, click **Yes, save these settings for this program**.

Getting Troubleshooting Help

If you can't solve a problem on your own, there are plenty of resources available to help you. In the next two sections, I show you how to get troubleshooting help online and by allowing another person to control your PC remotely.

Online Resources

The internet is home to an astonishingly wide range of information, but its forté has always been computer knowledge. Whatever problem you may have, there's a good chance that someone out there has run into the same thing, knows how to fix it, has posted the solution on a website or newsgroup, or would be willing to share the solution with you if asked. True, finding what you need is sometimes difficult—and you often can't be sure how accurate some of the solutions are. However, if you stick to the more reputable sites and get second opinions on solutions offered by complete strangers, then you'll find the online world an excellent troubleshooting resource. Here's my list of favorite online resources to check out:

- **Microsoft Product Support Services (support.microsoft.com)** This is Microsoft's main online technical support site. Through this site, you can access Windows 7 frequently asked questions (FAQs), see a list of known problems, download files, and send questions to Microsoft support personnel.

- **Microsoft Knowledge Base** The Microsoft Product Support Services site has links that enable you to search the Microsoft Knowledge Base, which is a database of articles related to all Microsoft products (including, of course, Windows 7). These articles provide you with information about Windows 7 and instructions on using Windows 7 features. But the most useful aspect of the Knowledge Base is for troubleshooting problems. Many of the articles were written by Microsoft support personnel after helping customers overcome problems. By searching for error codes or key words, you can often get specific solutions to your problems.

- **Vendor websites** All but the tiniest hardware and software vendors maintain websites with customer support sections that you can peruse for upgrades, patches, workarounds, FAQs, and sometimes a discussion board, which lets you talk to other users of the product.

The Remote Control Route

Here's a common troubleshooting scenario that you've probably come across a time or two. You notice a problem with your computer, try to fix it yourself, but to no avail. So you call up someone who knows about these things—it might be a son or daughter, one of your grandkids, a family friend, or a neighbor—and you explain the problem. The other person offers a few suggestions, but it's soon clear that he or she needs to be at your computer to troubleshoot the problem, so you end up with a vague promise to "take a look at it next time I'm over."

When it comes to tracking down and fixing computer woes, much of the time it's just too difficult unless you're sitting down in front of the machine where you can see exactly what's happening and then (hopefully) take specific steps to solve the problem.

Rather than waiting for someone to take a look at your computer the next time he or she comes to your house, you can have your would-be savior work with your computer right away, no matter where that person happens to be.

That sounds like magic, but it's entirely possible using a terrific feature called Windows Remote Assistance, which enables you to invite another person to connect to your computer over the internet. Once that connection is made, the other person can then see exactly what you see on your screen, and your friend can even take control of your computer temporarily to run troubleshooting and problem-solving steps.

Here's how it works:

1. Select **Start**, **All Programs**, **Maintenance**, **Windows Remote Assistance**.

2. Click **Invite someone you trust to help you**.

3. Click **Use e-mail to send an invitation**. Remote Assistance forges a new email message, as shown in Figure 6.5.

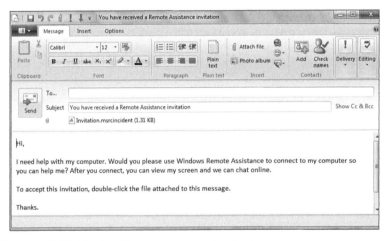

Figure 6.5: To invite someone to help you, you can send the invitation via email.

4. Type the address of the person you want to invite, then click **Send**. Remote Assistance then displays a connection password similar to the one shown in Figure 6.6.

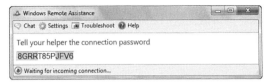

Figure 6.6: Remote Assistance generates a random password for your helper.

From here, your helper receives your email, opens the attached file, and is prompted for the password. At this point, you'd need to connect with the helper by phone to relay the password and allow the person to make the connection. When that happens, Remote Assistance asks you to confirm by displaying the dialog box shown in Figure 6.7. Click **Yes** to allow your helper to connect.

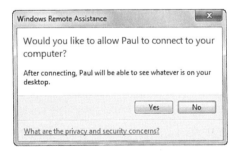

Figure 6.7: When your helper tries to connect, click **Yes** to allow it.

At this point, you can take your helper through whatever steps caused your problem, and hopefully he or she will provide sage advice. (Again, my assumption here is that the two of you are also talking on the phone at the same time.)

If your helper sees a solution to the problem, he or she can try explaining it to you—but these things almost always go a lot faster if the helper can just perform the fix. To do that, he or she clicks **Request control** in Remote Assistance, and you see the dialog box shown in Figure 6.8.

Activate the **Allow *Helper* to respond to User Account Control prompts** (where *Helper* is the name of the person helping you), then click **Yes**.

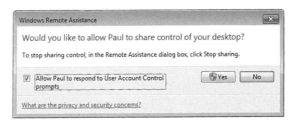

Figure 6.8: When your helper requests control of your computer, click **Yes**.

Recovering from a Problem

Solving a problem is one thing, but sometimes you have to mop up after the problem to restore your system to its previous state. This could be something as simple as restoring a lost file from a backup to reverting your entire system to a previous (presumably working) state. The rest of this chapter takes you through various recovery scenarios.

Recovering a Lost File

A system crash doesn't usually take any data down with it, but if a program crashes, the document you're working on may become corrupted or even disappear from your system entirely. Not good! If a document goes down for the count, Windows has got your back because you can recover the file from a recent backup. Here's how:

1. Select **Start**, **All Programs**, **Maintenance**, **Backup and Restore**. The Backup and Restore window appears.

2. Click **Restore my files**. The Restore Files wizard takes the stage.

3. Click **Search**.

4. In the Search For text box, type all or part of the name of the file, then click **Search**. The Restore Files wizard displays a list of files that match your typing.

5. Activate the check box beside the file you want to restore, as shown in Figure 6.9, and then click **OK**.

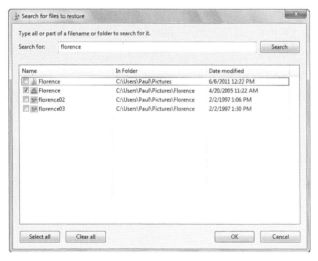

Figure 6.9: Run a search for your lost or corrupted file, and then activate its check box.

6. Click **Next**.

7. Click **Restore**.

8. If the Restore Files wizard tells you there is already a file with the same name, click **Copy and Replace**.

9. Click **Finish**.

Recovering from Program Crashes

If you've used Windows for any length of time, you'll be familiar with the fist-poundingly and hair-pullingly frustrating experience of the program crash. You're sailing along, doing whatever it is you do with the program in question, when suddenly it digs in its heels and refuses to go any further. You press all kinds of keys, click your mouse furiously, and hurl uncharitable suggestions at it—but the beast just sits there, frozen in its digital tracks.

How can you be sure that the program has crashed? The easiest way is to look at the program's title bar. If Windows can no longer communicate with the program normally, you'll see "Not Responding" in parentheses, as shown in Figure 6.10.

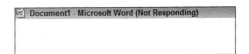

Figure 6.10: If you see "Not Responding" in the program's title bar, it almost always means that the program has crashed.

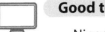

Good to Know!

Nine times out of ten the "Not Responding" text tells you the program has crashed. However, if the program is in the middle of a task that requires a lot of computing resources, it may not respond to Windows right away—and you'll see "Not Responding" in the title bar. To be certain, give the program a bit of time to complete any operations before declaring it dead in the water.

Before proceeding, you need to shut down the offending program before it causes system-wide instability or causes your other programs to run slowly. How do you shut down a program that refuses to respond? By using the Windows Task Manager, which you can access by using either of the following methods:

- Press **Ctrl+Alt+Delete** (this key combo is known whimsically as both the *three-fingered salute* and the *Vulcan nerve pinch*), then click **Start Task Manager**.

- Right-click some empty space on the taskbar, then click **Task Manager**.

You see a window similar to the one shown in Figure 6.11.

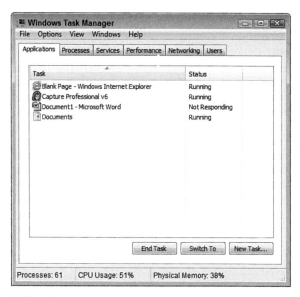

Figure 6.11: Task Manager lets you know if a program is non-responsive and, if so, lets you shut it down so you can move on with your life.

In the **Applications** tab, the **Task** column shows you a list of the programs you have running, and the **Status** column shows one of the following:

- **Running** This means that Windows can still communicate with the program. If your seemingly crashed program displays this status, it may mean that it's in the middle of a long or processor-intensive operation. You should wait a few minutes to give the program time to finish the operation.

- **Not Responding** This means that Windows can't get the program's attention, so it's official that the program has crashed.

If your program shows the "Not Responding" status or if it still shows "Running" after a few minutes, click the program to highlight it and then click **End Task**. Windows will then attempt to shut down the program in a civilized manner. If it isn't successful, you'll see a dialog box similar to the one shown in Figure 6.12. Click **Close the program** to tell Windows to stop messing around and just blow the darned program out of the water.

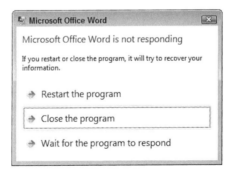

Figure 6.12: You see this dialog box if Windows can't shut down the stalled program via the usual channels.

Recovering Using System Restore

One of the most frustrating Windows experiences is your system sailing along without so much as an electronic hiccup, then having everything crash or become unstable after installing a program or a chunk of hardware. This all-too-common scenario means that some program component or device driver simply doesn't get along with your computer and that the two are now at loggerheads. Uninstalling the program or device can often help, but that's not a foolproof solution.

To help guard against software or hardware installations that bring down the system, Windows has a feature called System Protection. Its job is straightforward, yet clever: taking periodic snapshots—called *restore points*—of your system, each of which includes the current Windows 7 configuration. The idea is that if a program or device installation causes problems on your system, you use another feature called System Restore to revert your system to the most recent restore point before the installation.

System Protection automatically creates restore points as you work with your computer. For example, it creates a restore point every 24 hours if you keep your computer on full-time, and it also creates a restore point when you install software. This is great news, because it enables you to restore your entire system to a previous state and (hopefully!) get your system working again.

By the Way

If your computer won't start properly, you can still revert your system to a restore point. Start your computer, and immediately begin tapping the **F8** key until you see the Advanced Boot Options screen. Select **Safe Mode** in the list, then press **Enter**. When Windows loads, follow the steps in this section.

To revert your system to a restore point, close all your running programs, then follow these steps:

1. Select **Start**, **All Programs**, **Accessories**, **System Tools**, **System Restore**.

2. The first dialog box you see depends on your system. If you have no recent updates, the first dialog box just gives you an overview of System Restore, so click **Next**. Otherwise, the first dialog box gives you two options:

   - **Recommended restore**   Click this option to restore your system to the state it was in before the most recent update. This should work most of the time, so I recommend starting with this option. Click **Next**, and skip to step 5.

   - **Choose a different restore point**   Click this option if you know you want to use a different restore point or if you tried the most recent one and it didn't solve your problem. Click **Next**. The wizard conjures up the System Restore dialog box shown in Figure 6.13.

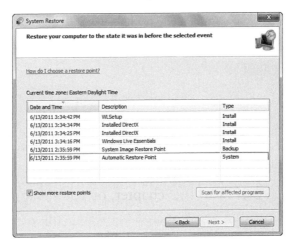

Figure 6.13: Use this window to choose the restore point you want to revert to.

3. Click the restore point you want to restore. (Note that the Automatic Restore Point items are the restore points created automatically by Windows 7 each time you start your computer.)

4. Click **Next**. System Restore displays a dialog box to confirm the restore point.

5. Click **Finish**. System Restore, apparently a paranoid little program, once again asks you to confirm.

6. Click **Yes**. System Restore begins restoring the restore point. When it's done, it restarts your computer.

7. If you see the System Restore dialog box telling you that the restore was successful, clap your hands excitedly and then click **Close**.

> **What Can Go Wrong?**
>
> Sometimes restoring your system makes things worse or causes additional problems. If that happens, you have a couple choices. To undo the restore, launch System Restore, click **Next**, select the **Restore Operation** restore point, and click **Next**. Alternatively, you can run System Restore and revert the system to an even earlier restore point.

Recovering Your System from a Backup

If worse comes to worst and you have to replace your computer's hard drive, you may think that all your documents and programs are lost. Not so—if your computer is backed up and you have a system repair disc, as discussed earlier in this chapter, or your Windows installation disc. That's because a Windows 7 backup includes a *system image*, which is geek-speak for "the whole shebang." This means you can restore the system image to your new hard drive, and all your documents, programs, and settings will also be restored.

Here are the steps to get started if you have a system repair disc:

1. Turn on (or restart) your computer.
2. Immediately after you turn on your computer, insert the system repair disc.
3. When you see the message, "Press any key to boot from CD/DVD...", press a key. System Recovery takes a minute or two to load.
4. Click **Next**. System Recovery Options prompts you to enter a username and password.
5. Type your Windows 7 username and password, then click **OK**.

Follow these steps to get started if you're using your Windows installation disc:

1. Turn on (or restart) your computer.
2. Immediately after you turn on your computer, insert the system repair disc.
3. When you see the message, "Press any key to boot from CD/DVD...", press a key.
4. Click **Next**.
5. Click **Repair your computer**.
6. Click **Next**.

Either way, the System Recovery Options dialog box appears, as shown in Figure 6.14.

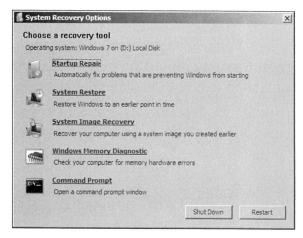

Figure 6.14: System Recovery Options offers a fine selection of recovery tools.

Make sure the external hard drive that you used for your backups is connected to your computer, then click **System Image Recovery**. In the Select a System Image Backup dialog box that appears, select **Use the latest system image** option, click **Next**, click **Next** again, and then click **Finish**. System Recovery restores your entire system (which takes a while—30 to 60 minutes).

The Least You Need to Know

- For easier recovery down the road, set up automatic backups and create a system repair disc.
- If a problem occurs soon after you changed something on your computer—a Windows setting, a program, a device, and so on—try reversing that change to see whether this fixes the error.

- You can often recover from problems just by shutting down all running programs, logging off Windows, or rebooting the computer.
- Take advantage of online resources such as Microsoft Product Support Services (particularly the Knowledge Base), vendor websites, and newsgroups (particularly the Google Groups search engine).
- To recover from a more serious problem, use System Restore to revert your system to an earlier (working) state.
- If your computer goes completely down for the count, you can restore everything by booting to a system repair disc or your Windows installation disc, then restoring the most recent system image.

Making Your Computer Easier to Use

Part 2

You'll be forgiven if, at this relatively early stage of your computing career, you believe that computers have been designed by and for young whippersnappers with 20/20 eyesight, bat-like hearing, and the nimbleness of a ballerina. Ah, that's because it's true! Why else would the screen type be so tiny, warning beeps all but inaudible, and the mouse a constant battle for control?

However, although right out of the box your computer presents a few too many challenges for older eyes, ears, and hands, there's no reason why it has to stay that way. In fact, the young guns who created Windows were also kind enough to load it to the brim with tools, features, and settings that can make your computer far *less* challenging. You can make text and images easier to see, sounds easier to hear, and the mouse and keyboard easier to use. The chapters in Part 2 tell you everything you need to know.

Circumventing Visual Challenges

Chapter 7

In This Chapter

- Making screen text and icons bigger
- Making screen items easier to see
- Getting rid of screen distractions
- Having screen text read aloud to you

Those of you who are no longer spring chickens (or even summer chickens, for that matter) know one thing for certain: the older you get, the worse your eyesight becomes. Sure, you can ramp up your eyeglass prescription or invest in extra-strength reading glasses—but even that may not be enough when it comes to reading text and deciphering icons on your computer screen. And, of course, if your eyesight problems go beyond simple afflictions such as farsightedness or astigmatism, then a change of eyewear isn't going to help you make sense of what's happening on your monitor.

Whatever the source of your visual challenges, you can't work with Windows if you can't see what Windows is trying to show you onscreen. Fortunately, you *can* put Windows to work making it easier to see text, icons, and images. As you will see in this chapter, Windows offers a number of tools for enlarging screen items, making things easier to see, reducing visual distractions, and even hearing audio translations of what's on the screen.

Making Things Bigger

If, like me, your 20/20 vision is available only in hindsight, you may be asking yourself a simple question: Why oh why does everything on my computer screen look so darned tiny? The icons are miniature, the buttons are minute, and the text is miniscule. It would be enough to drive a person to madness if these things were set in stone (electronically speaking, of course), but the good news is that they're not. As the next few sections show, Windows offers tools that can enlarge what you see on your screen. Your eyes will thank you.

Adjust the Screen Resolution

The reason why everything on your screen is positively pint-sized is because of the *screen resolution*, which determines the number of pixels used to display stuff on the screen. A *pixel* is an individual pinpoint of light, and all the colors you see on your screen are the result of thousands of these pixels getting turned on and set to display a specific hue.

An example screen resolution is 800 × 600, which means that Windows uses pixels arranged in a grid that has 800 columns and 600 rows. That's nearly half a million pixels for your viewing pleasure! However, a resolution of 1440 × 900 uses nearly 1.3 million pixels, so these things are relative.

Here's the key point: the more pixels you use, the *smaller* things will look on the screen. So if you're squinting like a fiend at your screen, it's likely because the screen resolution is set too high. Dial it back a bit, and things will get immediately easier to see because they'll be larger.

For example, Figure 7.1 shows the Windows 7 screen at 1440 × 900 resolution—which, as you can see, is barely readable. Now, contrast that with the screen shown in Figure 7.2, which uses 800 × 600 resolution. The difference is significant, to say the least.

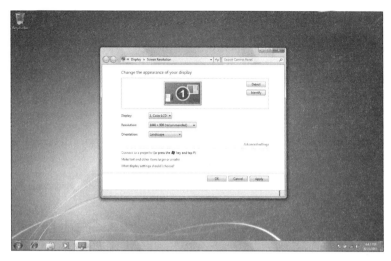

Figure 7.1: With a screen resolution of 1440 × 900, text and icons are microscopic.

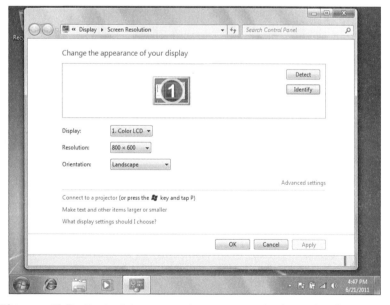

Figure 7.2: Switching to a lower resolution (in this case, all the way down to 800 × 600) makes everything much easier to see.

What Can Go Wrong?

You may be tempted to crank the resolution down to the lowest setting to get the largest version of the text and other screen items. However, that may cause problems because many Windows items are simply too big to fit into anything less than a 1024 × 768 screen.

Here's how you go about changing the screen resolution:

1. Select **Start**, **Control Panel** to open the Control Panel window.

2. Under the **Appearance and Personalization** heading, click **Adjust screen resolution**.

3. Click the **Resolution** list, then drag the slider to a lower resolution.

4. Click **Apply**. Windows changes the resolution and then asks whether you want to keep the new setting.

5. If you do, click **Keep changes**; otherwise, click **Revert** and repeat steps 3 and 4 until you get the resolution you prefer.

6. When you're done, click **OK**.

The Windows Vista steps for changing the screen resolution are the same as I've given here. For Windows XP, select **Start**, **Control Panel**, click **Appearance and Themes**, and then click **Change the screen resolution**.

Scale the Screen

Changing the screen resolution as I described in the previous section is a straightforward way to make things look bigger, but it suffers from a couple drawbacks:

- The lower the resolution, the bigger the screen text and images—but the greater the chance that something won't fit entirely on the screen.

- Higher screen resolutions display text and images sharply and crisply, but the lower the resolution you use, the more jagged and fuzzy the screen items appear—which can actually make them *less* readable.

So should you just go back to a higher resolution and buy more powerful reading glasses? Actually, there's a better way. Yes, you can switch to a higher screen resolution, but Windows offers another tool called *scaling* that can make both text and images appear larger while also preserving the sharpness that comes with the higher resolution. Win-win!

Let's look at an example. Figure 7.3 shows the Start menu on a system running at 800 × 600. Now, check out the Start menu in Figure 7.4, which was taken on a system running at 1440 × 900 but with scaling applied. As you can see, the latter is much sharper and easier to read.

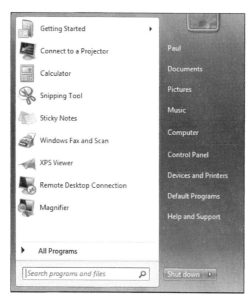

Figure 7.3: The Start menu with a screen resolution of 800 × 600.

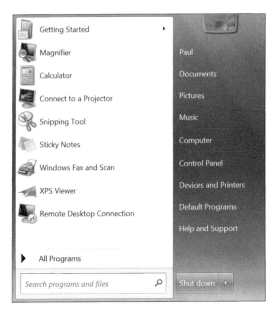

Figure 7.4: The Start menu with a screen resolution of 1400 × 900, scaled to a larger size.

To pull this off, first follow the steps from the previous section to set the screen resolution to one that's best for your monitor. How do you know which one is best? In the Resolution list, look for the one that says "Recommended."

Now, follow these steps to scale the screen:

1. Select **Start**, **Control Panel** to display the Control Panel.

2. Click **Appearance and Personalization**.

3. Under the **Display** heading, click **Make text and other items larger or smaller**.

4. If the items on your screen just need a little boost in size, click **Medium – 125%**, which makes everything 25 percent larger. If the items on your screen appear really teensy, then go for **Larger – 150%** instead.

5. Click **Apply**. Windows tells you that you have to log off to put the new setting into effect.

6. Click **Log off now**.

When you log back in, all the items on the screen will look bigger.

In Windows Vista, select **Start, Control Panel**, click **Optimize visual display**, and then click **Change the size of text and icons**. For Windows XP, select **Start, Control Panel**, click **Appearance and Themes, Change the screen resolution**, click **Advanced**, and then choose a value in the DPI Setting list.

Zoom In on the Screen

You may find that although you can make out most of the items on the screen, the occasional icon or bit of text is just too diminutive to decipher. One solution would be to increase the screen resolution or scaling, as I described in the previous two sections, but that seems like overkill.

You could always grab a nearby magnifying glass to get a closer look at the section you can't make out, but Windows offers an electronic version of the same thing. It's called—appropriately—Magnifier, and it enables you to temporarily zoom in on a portion of the screen.

To give Magnifier a whirl, select **Start, All Programs, Accessories, Ease of Access, Magnifier**. In the Magnifier window that appears, click **Views** and then click **Lens**, and click **Zoom in** (the **+** icon) until you get the magnification you want—and then move the mouse pointer over the area you want to magnify (the lens moves along with the mouse pointer). Figure 7.5 shows the Magnifier lens zoomed in on the WordPad ribbon.

Good to Know!

You can start Magnifier right from the keyboard. Press **Windows logo key+U** to open the Ease of Access center, then press **Alt+G**.

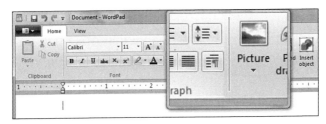

Figure 7.5: Use Magnifier's lens tool to enlarge parts of the screen.

Magnifier's even easier to use if you take advantage of the keyboard shortcuts listed in Table 7.1.

Table 7.1 Keyboard Shortcuts That Work with Magnifier

Press	To
Ctrl+Alt+F	Turn off the lens and see the full screen
Ctrl+Alt+L	Display the lens
Windows logo key+Plus sign (+)	Increase the magnification
Windows logo key+Minus sign (–)	Decrease the magnification

In Windows Vista, select **Start, All Programs, Accessories, Ease of Access, Magnifier.** For Windows XP, select **Start, All Programs, Accessories, Accessibility, Magnifier.**

Making Things Easier to See

Picking out certain items on the screen can often be a tough bit of business because Windows tends to display things in a jumble of icons, windows, dialog boxes, and other screen bric-a-brac. Things are made even worse if your eyesight is poor, because then you may find that it's next to impossible to distinguish screen objects such as the mouse pointer or the blinking cursor in a text program. Fortunately, Windows has solutions for these and similar problems, as the next few sections show.

Switch to a High-Contrast Screen

Windows tends to use fairly subtle colors that are designed not to overload your retinas with garish contrasts. However, sometimes Windows goes too far and displays, say, sky-blue text on a white background. That looks nice, sure, but boy can it be hard to read.

The solution is *more* contrast, not less. For example, black text on a white background, or white text on a black background. Windows actually comes with several high-contrast *themes*, which are collections of color schemes that apply all at once to text, windows, the desktop, and so on.

Follow these steps to apply a high-contrast theme:

1. Select **Start**, **Control Panel** to open the Control Panel.

2. Under **Appearance and Personalization**, click **Change the theme**. Control Panel opens the Personalization window.

3. In the list of themes, scroll to the bottom and then click the theme you want: High Contrast #1, High Contrast #2, High Contrast Black, or High Contrast White. Figure 7.6 shows the Personalization window with the High Contrast White theme applied.

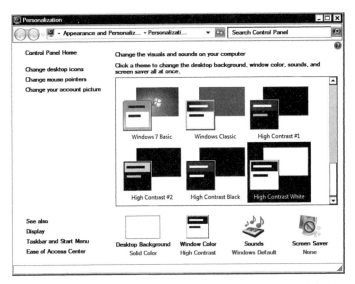

Figure 7.6: The Personalization window with the High Contrast White theme applied.

Good to Know!

You can switch between your regular theme and the high-contrast theme you chose in step 3 by pressing **Shift+Alt+Print Screen**. (Make sure you use the left Shift and left Alt keys for this.) When Windows asks you to confirm, click **Yes**.

In Windows Vista, select **Start, Control Panel, Appearance and Personalization**, and then under the Personalization heading, click **Change the theme**. In Windows XP, select **Start, Control Panel, Accessibility, Accessibility Options**, click the **Display** tab, activate the **Use High Contrast** check box, and then click **Settings** to configure the theme.

Make the Mouse Pointer Easier to See

That little white mouse pointer can be frustratingly difficult to pinpoint on a screen plastered with windows and text. To fix that, Windows offers several larger mouse pointers—and also *inverting* mouse pointers that change to a contrasting color as the mouse moves over different parts of the screen. Here's what you do:

1. Select **Start, All Programs, Accessories, Ease of Access, Ease of Access Center**. If you're in more of a keyboard mood, press **Windows logo key+U** instead.

2. Click **Make the mouse easier to use**.

3. Use the **Mouse pointers** box (see Figure 7.7) to click a pointer style that looks like it would be easy for you to pick out on the screen.

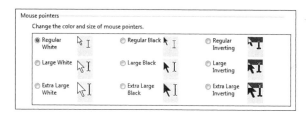

Figure 7.7: Use the Mouse pointers list to pick out an easier-to-see pointer.

4. Click **OK**.

If you're running Windows Vista, you can use the same steps to choose a mouse pointer. For Windows XP, select **Start, Control Panel, Appearance and Themes**, click **Mouse Pointers**, click the **Pointers** tab, and then use the **Scheme** list to choose one of the Large or Extra Large pointer schemes.

Make Dialog Boxes Easier to See

Dialog boxes are a fact of Windows life, and although they seem to pop up with alarming frequency, they're really a great feature because they let you know what Windows is up to and they enable you to tell Windows or a program exactly what you want done.

Unfortunately, dialog boxes are often busy with text and controls, such as check boxes, text boxes, and lists—so they can be hard to figure out. There are two cases where dealing with dialog boxes is particularly difficult:

- If you have trouble using a mouse, you can still navigate a dialog box by pressing the **Tab** key, which takes you from one control to the next. In geek-speak, this is known as changing which control has the *focus*. How do you know which control currently has the focus? Windows displays a rectangle around the control, but that rectangle can be hard to make out if your eyesight isn't the greatest.

- When you select a text box, Windows adds a vertical line inside the box, and that line tells you where the next character will appear. The line blinks on and off (so that you don't confuse it with, say, the letter *l* or the number *1*), but it's quite thin and therefore hard to see.

Windows offers a couple settings that can help solve both problems: it can make the focus rectangle thicker, and it can widen the blinking cursor. Follow these steps to configure one or both of these settings:

1. Select **Start, All Programs, Accessories, Ease of Access, Ease of Access Center.** Alternatively, press **Windows logo key+U.**

2. Click **Make the computer easier to see.**

3. To beef up the focus rectangle, activate the **Make the focus rectangle thicker** check box.

4. To widen the blinking cursor, click the **Set the thickness of the blinking cursor** list and then click the size you want to use. (The Preview box shows you an example.)

5. Click **OK**.

Figure 7.8 shows an example of the thicker focus rectangle.

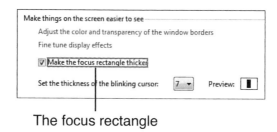

The focus rectangle

Figure 7.8: A thicker focus rectangle and blinking cursor can make dialog boxes a tad easier to use.

If you're running Windows Vista, you can use these same steps to configure the dialog box settings. Windows XP only supports changing the blinking cursor width. Select **Start, Control Panel, Accessibility, Accessibility Options**, click the **Display** tab, and then adjust the **Width** slider.

Removing Distractions

Sometimes it's difficult to get a good look at an item on the screen—not because the item itself is hard to see but because something else on the screen is getting in the way. Perhaps the best example is a desktop background that sports a busy, multicolored design that makes the item you're *supposed* to be looking at difficult to even locate on the screen.

Another example is the collection of animation effects that Windows uses. For example, when you minimize a window, it "shrinks" down to its taskbar icon. Similarly, pull-down menus appear to slide down from the menu bar, and program windows fade in when you open them and fade out when you close them. These are harmless effects most of the time—but not if they distract your gaze from something else and you have trouble finding it again.

If either or both of these features are driving you to distraction, follow these steps to turn them off:

1. Select **Start, All Programs, Accessories, Ease of Access, Ease of Access Center.** You can also press **Windows logo key+U.**

2. Click **Make the computer easier to see**.

3. To nix the animation effects, activate the **Turn off all unnecessary animations** check box.

4. To block the background, activate the **Remove background images** check box.

5. Click **OK** to put the new settings into effect.

If you're running Windows Vista, the steps for turning off these features are exactly the same. In Windows XP, to turn off animation effects select **Start**, right-click **My Computer**, click **Properties**, click the **Advanced** tab, click **Settings** in the Performance group, and then select the **Adjust for best performance** option.

Hearing What's on the Screen

If you find that you're really having trouble making out what's on the screen, Windows comes with an assistive technology called Narrator that can help. Narrator's job is to read aloud whatever text appears in the current window or dialog box. Narrator also does many other things, including the following:

- Tells you the name of the current window or dialog box and lists the contents of that window or dialog box
- Tells you the name of the dialog box control that currently has the focus, the type of control (for example, a check box), and the control's current state (for example, checked)
- Echoes your most recent keystroke. For example, if you press Tab to move to the next dialog box control, Narrator says "Tab."
- Tells you the text of the selected link in Internet Explorer

By the Way

Narrator isn't perfect. It has trouble with unusual words that aren't in its database (for example, it pronounces *iPhone* as *ee-FUN-ee*); it can sometimes take a few seconds to convert all the text in a window or dialog box to speech, so some patience is required; and it can take a while to get used to how the program works. Still, it's better than not knowing what's happening on the screen.

If you're ready to give Narrator a go, press **Windows logo key+U** to open the Ease of Access center, then press **Alt+N**.

Use the same technique to open Narrator in Windows Vista. To start Narrator in Windows XP, select **Start, All Programs, Accessories, Accessibility, Narrator**. From the keyboard, press **Windows logo key, P, Enter, A, Enter, N, Enter**.

First off, you may want to configure some Narrator settings:

- **Slowing down the speech.** If you find that Narrator talks a bit too fast, you can slow it down. Press **Alt+V** to choose the **Voice Settings** button, press **Alt+S** to select the **Set Speed** list, and then press **Down arrow**. Narrator will tell you each new value (the default speed is five). Try three or four, then press **Enter** to exit the dialog box.

- **Starting Narrator minimized.** If you find the Narrator window is taking up too much of the screen, you can press **Alt+Spacebar** and then **N** to minimize it. If you want to start Narrator minimized, press **Alt+Z** to activate the **Start Narrator Minimized** check box.

- **Starting Narrator when you start Windows.** If you want Narrator to run automatically each time you launch Windows, press **Tab** until you hear Narrator tell you that the **Control whether Narrator starts when I log on** hyperlink is selected, then press **Enter**. Now, press **Alt+U** to activate the **Turn on Narrator** check box. Press **Tab** until Narrator tells you that the **OK** button is selected, then press **Enter**.

The Least You Need to Know

- One way to make items look larger on your screen is to switch to a lower screen resolution.
- To make things bigger onscreen *and* keep text and icons sharp, use the screen resolution recommended for your monitor and use a higher scaling percentage.
- A quick way to open the Ease of Access Center is to press **Windows logo key+U**.
- You can use Magnifier to zoom in on sections of the screen. Select **Start**, **All Programs**, **Accessories**, **Ease of Access**, **Magnifier**.
- You can make things easier to see onscreen by switching to a high-contrast color scheme and using larger mouse pointers.
- To get Windows to read screen text and keystrokes aloud, start Narrator by pressing **Windows logo key+U** and then **Alt+N**.

Chapter 8

Surmounting Hearing Challenges

In This Chapter

- Deciding whether to use speakers or headphones
- Turning up the volume for the entire system and for individual programs
- Adjusting headphone volume for your left and right ears
- Smoothing audio to avoid wide fluctuations in volume
- Displaying visual cues each time Windows or a program makes a sound

From your perspective as a user, computers are mostly visual contraptions. That is, whether you're typing text, using the mouse, or navigating a menu system, what you see onscreen is the important thing. However, as you've seen, computer communication is a two-way street—so not only do you provide input to the computer, but it also provides feedback that lets you know what's happening and whether it needs more information from you. This feedback is mostly visual—dialog boxes, notifications, and the like—but it's not *entirely* visual. Often, your computer will try to catch your attention by beeping or making some other sound to let you know something's happening.

And, of course, your computer is fully capable of making more interesting sounds, such as those you hear when you play music, videos, and movies.

If your hearing has deteriorated over the years, or if you have a hearing impairment in one or both ears, detecting system sounds and enjoying music and movies can be a challenge. Fortunately, help is at hand. There are some devices you can use to make it easier to hear computer sound, and Windows has a few tools that you can configure to help or work around your hearing issues. This chapter gives you the low-down on the hi-fi.

Speakers or Headphones?

If you suffer from only minor hearing loss, you may be able to compensate by turning up the volume of your computer speakers (as I describe in the next section). However, this may be impractical if there are other people nearby and you don't want to disturb them.

In such cases, an often better solution is to replace the speakers with headphones. Because the sound from the headphones takes a shorter and more direct path to your ear, it can make the sounds sharper and easier to discern—and it has the added advantage of not disturbing anyone within earshot.

If you decide to invest in some headphones, here are a few pointers to bear in mind:

- If you use an in-the-ear (ITE) hearing aid, look for ear-pad headphones (also called on-ear headphones), which rest on your ears.

- If you use a behind-the-ear (BTE) hearing aid, you'll need to move up to full-size headphones (also called full-cup, ear-cup, or over-the-ear headphones), which are large enough to cover not only your ear but also your hearing aid microphone.

- With any type of hearing aid, you need to guard against feedback—that is, amplified sounds from your hearing aid "leaking" out and bouncing off the headphones back into the hearing aid. The cycle repeats until a painful feedback squeal is the result. To prevent this, get headphones that use foam ear pads, which reduce the chance of sounds being reflected into the hearing aid.

- If your hearing aid comes with a telecoil mode (which enables the hearing aid to process sounds sent electromagnetically), be sure to get telecoil-compatible headphones (which broadcast sounds electromagnetically).

- Consider getting noise-canceling headphones, which virtually eliminate background noises to let you hear just the sounds from the headphones.

Good to Know!

If you go the telecoil-compatible route for your headphones, be sure to activate your hearing aid's telecoil mode.

Once you have your headphones, in most cases you connect the headphone jack to the Line Out port on the back (or sometimes the front) of your computer (see my description for connecting speakers in Chapter 1). However, many headphones now connect via USB, so in that case you'd connect your headphones to a free USB port (again, see Chapter 1 for details).

Adjusting the Volume

Depending on the nature of your hearing impairment, the most straightforward solution would be to turn up the volume on your speakers or headphones. However, Windows also gives you more subtle ways to adjust the volume, such as turning up just a particular application, balancing headphone volume between the left and right speakers, and equalizing the volume to avoid wide fluctuations in loudness. The next few sections tell all.

Adjust the Overall System Volume

The *system volume* is the volume that Windows uses for all things audio on your computer: the sounds that Windows itself makes (warning beeps, the logon and logoff tones, and so on) and the sounds that waft from your applications (such as music from Media Player and the new-mail notification from Windows Live Mail).

To control the system volume, click the **Volume** icon in the taskbar's notification area to open the Volume control. (The icon looks like a speaker with sound waves coming out; see Figure 8.1.) Use your mouse to drag the slider up to the volume level you prefer. When you're done, close the Volume control either by pressing **Esc** or by clicking the desktop.

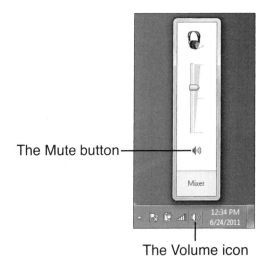

Figure 8.1: Click the **Volume** icon and then drag the slider to set the system volume.

Adjust an Application's Volume

Adjusting the system volume is the easiest way to get the sound level you need, but in many cases it's not the best way. For example, suppose that you're waiting for an important email message, so you set up Windows Live Mail to play a sound when an email message arrives. Suppose further that you're also using Windows Media Player to play music in the background. If you get a phone call, you have two choices:

- Turn down the music by using the Volume control to lower the system volume.
- Mute the music by clicking the Volume control's **Mute** button (pointed out in Figure 8.1).

However, turning down or muting the music playback also means turning down or muting other system sounds, including your email program's audio alerts. So while you're on the phone, there's a good chance that you'll miss that important message you've been waiting for.

Windows 7 (as well as Windows Vista) solves this problem by giving you control over the volume for *each* application that plays audio. Using a tool called the Volume Mixer, Windows gives you a volume-control slider for every running program that is either a dedicated sound application (such as Windows Media Player) or is currently producing audio output. In our example, you'd have separate volume controls for Windows Media Player and Windows Live Mail. When that phone call comes in, you can turn down or mute Windows Media Player while leaving the Windows Mail volume as is—so there's much less chance that you'll miss that incoming message.

By the Way

I'm sorry to report that Windows XP doesn't offer the Volume Mixer or anything similar.

To control the volume of an application, follow these steps:

1. Click the **Volume** icon in the taskbar's notification area. Windows displays the Volume control.

2. Click **Mixer**. Windows opens the Volume Mixer, which will appear similar to the one shown in Figure 8.2. (You'll definitely see the Device and System Sounds volume controls, but the rest will depend on which applications you're currently running and whether those applications are making sounds.)

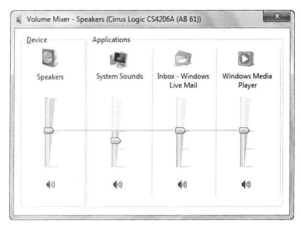

Figure 8.2: Use the Volume Mixer to adjust the volume of individual sound applications on your computer.

3. In the **Applications** area, use your mouse to drag the slider of the application you want to adjust.

4. Repeat step 3 for any other applications you want to mess with.

5. When you're done, click the red **Close** button (the "X") in the upper-right corner of the Volume Mixer window.

Balance Your Headphones

Sometimes, hearing troubles in one ear are particularly bad. Adjusting the system volume or an application's volume is problematic in these cases, because turning up the sound enough to hear things in your bad ear can make those sounds too loud in your other ear.

Windows can help by enabling you to balance the sound in each ear. That is, you can turn up the sound for your bad ear and/or turn down the sound for your good ear. Here's what you do:

1. Select **Start**, **Control Panel**, **Hardware and Sound**, **Sound**. Windows displays the Sound dialog box.

2. In the **Playback** tab, click **Headphones**.

> **By the Way**
>
> Depending on the type of headphones you're using, you might not see a Headphones item in the Playback tab. If not, look for a Speakers item where the description uses the word "Headset" (for example, Logitech USB Headset).

3. Click **Properties**.

4. Click the **Levels** tab.

5. Click **Balance**. Windows displays the Balance dialog box shown in Figure 8.3.

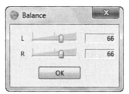

Figure 8.3: Use the Balance dialog box to adjust the headphone volume for each ear.

6. Use your mouse to drag the **L** (left) and **R** (right) sliders to the volume levels you prefer. (In some cases, instead of L you see the number 1, and instead of R you see the number 2.)

7. Click **OK** to put the new levels into effect and return to the Levels tab.

8. Click **OK**.

If you have Windows Vista, the steps for balancing headphone volume are identical to the ones I give here. If you have Windows XP, select **Start, Control Panel, Sounds, Speech, and Audio Devices**. Click **Change the speaker settings**, click **Speaker Volume**, use the **Left** and **Right** sliders to set the volume levels, and then click **OK**.

Equalize the Volume

For certain types of hearing impairments, wide fluctuations in volume can make sounds—particularly speech—much harder to perceive. You can compensate by turning on the Loudness Equalization enhancement for your computer's speakers or your headphones, which makes all sounds that emanate from your computer equally loud.

Follow these steps to turn on Loudness Equalization:

1. Select **Start, Control Panel, Hardware and Sound, Sound**. Windows displays the Sound dialog box.

2. In the **Playback** tab, click the sound device you use: **Speakers** or **Headphones**.

3. Click **Properties**.

4. Click the **Enhancements** tab.

5. Activate the **Loudness Equalization** check box, as shown in Figure 8.4.

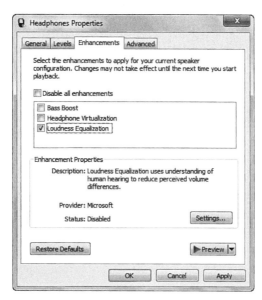

Figure 8.4: With the Loudness Equalization feature on the job, sounds such as speech will be easier to discern.

6. Click **OK**.

The Windows Vista steps for turning on Loudness Equalization are the same as I've given here. Unfortunately, Windows XP doesn't support this feature.

Getting Visual Cues to Screen Activity

If your hearing is impaired but your eyesight is fine, you can configure your computer to produce some sort of visual display for actions that are normally only accompanied by a sound. As the rest of this chapter shows, you can set up visual cues for system sounds, spoken dialog, and system notification messages.

Turn On Visual Notifications for Sounds

Many of the sounds emitted by your computer happen in the background. For example, you may be composing a letter in WordPad and Windows Live Mail beeps when a new email message arrives. Nothing else happens on the screen, so if you happen to not hear the beep, you won't know that you have new mail.

Anybody can have these background beeps go in one ear and out the other, but if your hearing is impaired, you stand that much more of a chance to miss what is often a fairly subtle sound. To ensure this isn't the case, you can activate the Sound Sentry feature. Sound Sentry displays a visual indicator each time your system makes a sound. By default, Sound Sentry flashes the title bar of the application that made the sound, but you can configure Sound Sentry to flash the entire window or flash the desktop.

Follow these steps to activate and configure Sound Sentry:

1. Select **Start**, **All Programs**, **Accessories**, **Ease of Access**, **Ease of Access Center**. For faster service, you can also press **Windows logo key+U**.

2. Click **Use text or visual alternatives for sounds**.

3. Activate the **Turn on visual notifications for sounds (Sound Sentry)** check box, as shown in Figure 8.5.

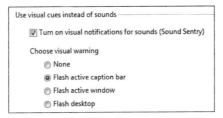

Figure 8.5: Activate Sound Sentry to see a visual cue whenever a program makes a sound.

4. In the **Choose visual warning** option group, choose **Flash active caption bar** (*caption bar* is another term for *title bar*), **Flash active window**, or **Flash desktop**. If you're not sure, stick with flashing the title bar. If that proves to be too subtle, try flashing the application window—and if you still need a bigger cue, go with flashing the desktop.

5. Click **OK**.

Follow the same steps to activate Sound Sentry in Windows Vista. In Windows XP, select **Start, Control Panel, Accessibility Options, Accessibility Options**, click the **Sound** tab, activate the **Use SoundSentry** check box, select an item from the **Choose the visual warning** list, and then click **OK**.

Display Text Captions for Spoken Dialog

Some applications include spoken dialog, which may be instructions for using the program or perhaps a welcome message. If those programs are also kind enough to include text captions for that dialog box (think Closed Captioning for the computer), then you can configure Windows to display that text while the dialog plays:

1. Select **Start, All Programs, Accessories, Ease of Access, Ease of Access Center**. If you're feeling a bit lazy, skip all that and just press **Windows logo key+U**.

2. Click **Use text or visual alternatives for sounds**.

3. Activate the **Turn on text captions for spoken dialog** check box, as shown in Figure 8.6.

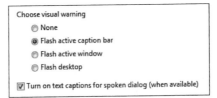

Figure 8.6: You can have Windows display text captions (when they're available) for spoken dialog.

4. Click **OK**.

Windows Vista users can follow the same steps to activate text captions. If you're a Windows XP user, select **Start**, **Control Panel**, **Accessibility Options**, **Accessibility Options**, click the **Sound** tab, activate the **Use ShowSounds** check box, and then click **OK**.

The Least You Need to Know

- If you opt to use headphones, get a pair that works best with either ITE or BTE hearing aids, has foam pads to prevent feedback, and is telecoil-compatible.
- Click the **Volume** icon in the notification area to adjust the system volume, and click **Mixer** to adjust the volume of individual applications.
- To balance your headphones, select **Start**, **Control Panel**, **Hardware and Sound**, **Sound**, click your headphones, click **Properties**, click **Levels**, and then click **Balance**.
- To equalize loudness, select **Start**, **Control Panel**, **Hardware and Sound**, **Sound**, click your speakers or headphones, click **Properties**, click **Enhancements**, and then activate **Loudness Equalization**.
- To activate Sound Sentry or text captions, select **Start**, **All Programs**, **Accessories**, **Ease of Access**, **Ease of Access Center** (or press **Windows logo key+U**), and then click **Use text or visual alternatives for sounds**.

Overcoming Physical Challenges

Chapter

9

In This Chapter

- Domesticating your mouse
- Controlling your keyboard
- Convincing notifications to stay onscreen for longer
- Going hands-free with voice commands

Using a computer may seem at first blush to be more of a mental exercise. After all, it seems as though you spend lots of time in front of the screen reading things, looking at things, and thinking about things.

However, if you mapped out your computer time, you'd almost certainly find that you spend great chunks of time on *physical* tasks: using your keyboard to press keys and type longer passages and using your mouse to point at, click, double-click, and drag things—not to mention whatever gesticulations and hands-on techniques that you use to cajole your computer into behaving sensibly for a change.

This surprisingly physical side of computing means that if you have physical challenges of your own, you may find it hard to perform certain tasks (and a few may be pretty much mission impossible). Fortunately, it doesn't have to be that way. Windows is loaded with tools and programs that either make using the mouse and keyboard less of a burden or that enable you to work around these devices altogether. This chapter tells you everything you need to know.

Making the Mouse Easier to Use

When you think about it, the mouse is an oddly contradictory piece of technology. On the one hand, you move this plastic lump on your desk and a little pointer on the screen moves at more or less the same time (and in a more or less comprehensible direction, once you get used to the fact that forward-and-back mouse movements translate to up-and-down pointer movements on the screen).

On the other hand, when it comes time to actually make the mouse do something useful, exquisite precision is required. Despite the fact that the tiniest movement of the mouse can send the pointer scooting across the screen, you're regularly asked to position the pointer over an impossibly small button or bit of text—and then, without moving the mouse in the slightest, you're supposed to click, double-click, or right-click that teensy target.

That's a tough row to hoe for even the most dexterous among us, but it becomes a major obstacle for anyone who has physical challenges that make such precise mouse movements a near impossibility. Fortunately, Windows comes with a few accessibility features that enable you to either forego the mouse altogether or have a bit more mouse leeway. The next few sections provide the particulars.

Control the Mouse Pointer with Your Keyboard

It's a fact of computing life that Windows has been designed from the ground up to be a mouse-centric system. Sure, there are keyboard shortcuts and techniques galore—but many things simply have no keyboard equivalent and require a mouse.

I should say that some things have no keyboard equivalent *unless* you take advantage of a Windows feature called *Mouse Keys*, which enables you to move the mouse pointer by using the arrow keys on the keyboard's numeric keypad. (These are the numbered keys arranged in three rows and three columns on the right side of your keyboard.) That is, you press the up arrow (the 8 key) to move the mouse up, the left arrow (the 4 key) to move the mouse left, and so on. Many people find this much easier than trying to maneuver the mouse into and out of tight screen spots.

By the Way

For Mouse Keys to work, make sure that you have your keyboard's Num Lock feature turned on. On most keyboards, you should see a light over or near the Num Lock key. If you don't see a light, press **Num Lock**. Note, too, that Mouse Keys doesn't work with the separate arrow-key-only keypads found on most modern keyboards.

Follow these steps to activate Mouse Keys:

1. Select **Start**, **Control Panel**, **Ease of Access**, **Change how your mouse works**. The Make the Mouse Easier to Use window appears on the desktop.

2. Activate the **Turn on Mouse Keys** check box, as shown in Figure 9.1.

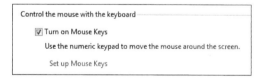

Figure 9.1: Activate Mouse Keys to control the mouse pointer from your keyboard.

3. Click **OK**.

Follow the same steps to activate Mouse Keys in Windows Vista. In Windows XP, select **Start, Control Panel, Accessibility Options, Accessibility Options**, click the **Mouse** tab, activate the **Use MouseKeys** check box, and then click **OK**.

Table 9.1 provides a complete list of what each numeric keypad key does while Mouse Keys is activated.

Table 9.1 Numeric Keypad Keys to Use with the Mouse Keys Feature

Press	To
1	Move the mouse pointer diagonally down and left
2	Move the mouse pointer down
3	Move the mouse pointer diagonally down and right
4	Move the mouse pointer left
5	Click
6	Move the mouse pointer right
7	Move the mouse pointer up and left
8	Move the mouse pointer up
9	Move the mouse pointer diagonally up and right
+	Double-click
/	Select the left mouse button
*	Select both mouse buttons
–	Select the right mouse button
Insert	Lock the selected button
Delete	Release the selected button

Here's how you use these keys:

- To click an object, use the arrow keys to move the pointer over the object, press the slash key (/) to select the left mouse button (if it isn't selected already), and press **5** to click.

Good to Know!

How do you know which mouse button is currently selected? When you activate Mouse Keys, Windows adds a mouse icon to the notification area. It indicates the currently selected button by marking the equivalent button on the mouse icon. In Windows 7, click the **notification area arrow**, click **Customize**, use the Mouse Keys list to select **Show icon and notifications**, and then click **OK**.

- To double-click an object, use the arrow keys to move the pointer over the object, press the slash key (/) to select the left mouse button, and press the plus sign (+) to double-click.

- To right-click an object, use the arrow keys to move the pointer over the object, press the minus sign (–) to select the right mouse button, and press **5**.

- To drag and drop an object, use the arrow keys to move the pointer over the object, press the slash key (/) to select the left mouse button, press **Insert** to lock the button, use the arrow keys to move the object to its destination, and press **Delete** to release the button and drop the object.

- To right-drag and drop an object, use the arrow keys to move the pointer over the object; press the minus sign (–) to select the right mouse button; press **Insert** to lock the button; use the arrow keys to move the object to its destination; and then press **Delete** to release the button, drop the object, and display the context menu.

The Need for Speed: Making Mouse Keys Faster

The first thing you'll notice about using Mouse Keys is that it is *slow*. You press and hold an arrow key with all your might, and the mouse pointer takes what can only be described as a leisurely stroll across the screen. Of course, you may not *want* the mouse pointer flying hither and yon—but if you'd like to pick up the pace, Windows is happy to help.

In the Make the Mouse Easier to Use window, click the **Set up Mouse Keys** link to bring up the Set up Mouse Keys window. In the **Pointer speed** section, shown in Figure 9.2, use the **Top speed** slider to set the maximum speed the mouse pointer moves when you hold down an arrow key. To speed things up, configure this setting closer to the **High** end of the scale. You can also use the **Acceleration** slider to specify how quickly the mouse pointer achieves its top speed after you hold down an arrow key. Again, drag the slider toward the **Fast** end of the scale for a speed boost.

Finally, I also recommend that you activate the **Hold down CTRL to speed up and SHIFT to slow down** check box. This means that you can hold down the **Ctrl** key to make the mouse pointer travel faster when you're holding down an arrow key. (Or, to slow down the pointer, you can hold down **Shift**.)

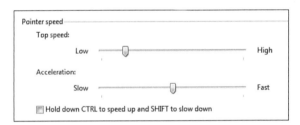

Figure 9.2: Use the settings in the Pointer speed group to turbocharge the Mouse Keys feature.

Easier Mouse Dragging

You probably know the mouse dragging drill by now: place the pointer over the object, press and hold the left mouse button, move the object to its new destination, and release the mouse button. If your mouse hand doesn't have much flexibility or mobility these days, then the idea of pressing and holding the left mouse button while you drag something is likely not very appealing (and may even be downright impossible).

The solution (you just *knew* there was going to be a solution, didn't you?) is a terrific feature called *ClickLock*. Rather than holding down the mouse button for the full extent of a drag (bad), you can "lock" the button into place for as long as you need it "held down," then unlock it when you're done (good).

Follow these steps to turn on this useful feature:

1. Select **Start, Control Panel, Hardware and Sound**.
2. Under the **Devices and Printers** heading, click **Mouse**.
3. Select the **Buttons** tab (if it isn't selected already).
4. Activate the **Turn on ClickLock** check box, as shown in Figure 9.3.

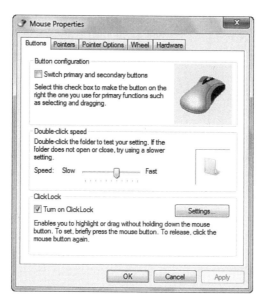

Figure 9.3: Activate ClickLock to drag stuff without having to hold down the mouse button.

5. Click **OK**.

With ClickLock on duty, move the mouse pointer over the object you want to drag, then press and hold the left mouse button for a couple seconds. This locks the mouse button (figuratively speaking; the button itself doesn't stay pressed), and you can now let go of the button and drag the object to and fro. When you're done, click the mouse button to release the lock.

In Windows Vista, select **Start**, **Control Panel**, **Mouse** and then follow steps 3 through 5. In Windows XP, select **Start, Control Panel, Printers and Other Hardware, Mouse**, and then follow steps 3 through 5.

Easier Window Selection

When you need to switch to another window, the standard method is to click the window's taskbar button. That works fine, but if your dexterity isn't what it used to be, it can sometimes be a long haul to get the mouse all the way down to the taskbar and then all the way back to the program window. Also, every now and then a program will have multiple windows on the go, in which case a second click is required to choose the window you want from the list that appears.

When switching windows, there's an easy way to avoid long mouse moves and multiple clicks: if you can see the window you want, click anywhere inside that window. Nice!

However, if you want this process to be even easier, Windows is up to the task. You can configure your system so that you switch to a window simply by placing the mouse pointer anywhere inside that window. No clicking required! Here's how to set this up:

1. Select **Start, All Programs, Accessories, Ease of Access, Change how your mouse works**.

2. Click to check the **Activate a window by hovering over it with the mouse** check box, as shown in Figure 9.4.

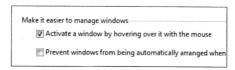

Figure 9.4: Check the **Activate a window ...** check box for clickless window switching.

3. Click **OK**.

If you're using Windows Vista, you can follow these same steps to turn on this setting.

By the Way

Alas, Windows XP doesn't support this handy feature.

Prevent Automatic Window Arranging

One of the features that debuted in Windows 7 is automatic window arranging:

- Drag a window to the left edge of the screen (technically, you have to drag until the mouse pointer reaches the left edge of the screen), and Windows 7 automatically arranges the window so that it takes up the left half of the desktop, as shown in Figure 9.5.

178 **Part 2:** Making Your Computer Easier to Use

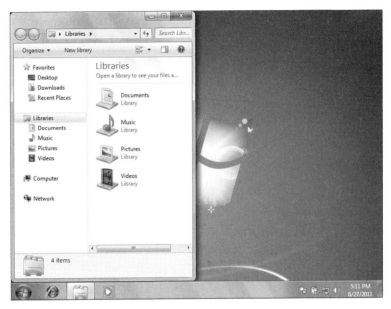

Figure 9.5: Drag a window to the left edge of the screen, and Windows 7 automatically arranges it to take up the left half of the desktop.

- Similarly, drag a window to the right edge of the screen and Windows 7 automatically arranges it to take up the right half of the desktop.
- Drag a window to the top edge of the screen, and Windows automatically maximizes the window when you release the mouse button.

These can be handy shortcuts, but if you're having trouble controlling the mouse, it can be supremely annoying to have Windows automatically arrange a window when you don't want it to. If this has happened to you one too many times, fight back by turning off this feature:

1. Select **Start, All Programs, Accessories, Ease of Access, Change how your mouse works**.

2. Activate the **Prevent windows from being automatically arranged when moved to the edge of the screen** check box, as shown in Figure 9.6.

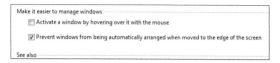

Figure 9.6: Activate the **Prevent windows from being automatically arranged ...** check box to put the kibosh on automatic window arranging.

3. Click **OK**.

> **By the Way**
>
> Because automatic window arranging is new to Windows 7, you won't be surprised to hear that Windows Vista and Windows XP don't have anything similar.

Making the Keyboard Easier to Use

If your first encounter with a mouse caused an excessive amount of brow-furrowing, chances are your brow remained smooth when you first laid your eyes and hands on a keyboard. It's a somewhat typewriter-ish device, so it's immediately familiar—and its purpose, typing letters and numbers (I'm ignoring the less comprehensible keys such as F1 and Ctrl here), is fairly straightforward.

But that doesn't mean the keyboard is easy to use, particularly for people who have mobility and dexterity challenges. For example, those keys can be awfully small targets, and I don't know who the sadist was who came up with key combinations such as Ctrl+Esc and Alt+Shift+Tab that would tax even the longest-fingered pianist.

Over the next few sections, I'll take you on a tour of the Windows features that can help solve these and other keyboard conundrums.

Press Multiple-Key Commands One Key at a Time

Keyboard shortcuts are a big part of Windows because much of the time, it's just easier and faster to keep your hands near the keyboard rather than reaching for the mouse. There are lots of single-key shortcuts in Windows: F1 for help, F2 to rename a file or folder, the Windows logo key to open the Start menu, and so on.

However, there are only so many of these "extra" keys to go around, so Windows gets around that limitation by using key combinations: Alt+Tab to switch windows, Ctrl+C to copy something, Ctrl+S to save something, and so on. Keys such as Ctrl, Alt, and Shift that Windows uses in these key combinations are called *modifier keys*, and the vast majority of keyboard shortcuts use a modifier key (and sometimes two!).

> **Definition**
>
> A **modifier key** is a key such as Ctrl, Alt, or Shift that you hold down while you press another key, such as a letter, number, or function key, to create a key combination.

The glaring problem here is that even a key combination involving two relatively nearby keys (such as Ctrl+C or Ctrl+V) can be extremely difficult to pull off for anyone whose hands simply don't want to bend that way. One alternative is to use one hand to hold down the modifier key and then use your other hand to press the second key.

That works, but it still requires you to hold down a key for a while. If you have trouble doing that, then you need to turn to Windows for help. In this case, help arrives in the form of a feature called *Sticky Keys*. When Sticky Keys is on, you can press a modifier key (such as Ctrl, Alt, Shift, or any combination of these), and the key remains active until you press another key. For example, to use the Ctrl+S key combination, you'd press **Ctrl** and then you'd press **S**. Note as well that Windows beeps each time you press a modifier key.

Follow these steps to activate Sticky Keys:

1. Select **Start, Control Panel, Ease of Access, Change how your keyboard works**. The Make the keyboard easier to use window appears.

2. Activate the **Turn on Sticky Keys** check box, as shown in Figure 9.7.

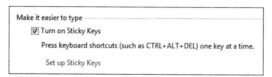

Figure 9.7: Activate Sticky Keys to press key combinations one key at a time.

3. Click **OK**.

Follow the same steps to activate Sticky Keys in Windows Vista. In Windows XP, select **Start, Control Panel, Accessibility Options, Accessibility Options**, click the **Keyboard** tab, activate the **Use StickyKeys** check box, and then click **OK**.

Sticky Situations: Sharing Your Computer

If you share your computer with another person, that person may not want to use Sticky Keys. To preserve harmony, it's possible to use Sticky Keys and regular key combinations on the same computer—just not at the same time. Let's see how this works.

By default, when the other person presses a regular key combination (such as Ctrl+C), Windows automatically turns off Sticky Keys so the other person can use the computer without having to worry about anything.

What about you? Does this mean you have to go through the steps in the previous section every time you sit down to the computer? Nope. By default, if you press the **Shift** key five times, Windows displays a dialog box asking whether you want to turn on Sticky Keys, and by clicking **Yes** you reactivate Sticky Keys.

What Can Go Wrong?

The press-the-Shift-key-five-times shortcut actually toggles Sticky Keys on and off. So if you don't see the dialog box, it means you actually turned Sticky Keys off. Whoops! In that case, just press **Shift** another five times to turn Sticky Keys back on.

To make sure both of these options are working, open the Make the Keyboard Easier to Use window and then click the **Set up Sticky Keys** link to display the Set up Sticky Keys window. As shown in Figure 9.8, make sure that the **Turn on Sticky Keys when SHIFT is pressed five times** check box and the **Turn off Sticky Keys when two keys are pressed at once** check box are activated.

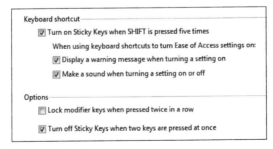

Figure 9.8: Use the Set up Sticky Keys window to customize the Sticky Keys feature.

Avoid Unwanted Keystrokes

If you want to enter a key multiple times, you can simply tap the key as many times as you need. However, it's a standard feature on all keyboards that when you press and hold a key, Windows assumes you want to enter that key multiple times. Windows first accepts the initial keystroke and then waits briefly (about half a second) to see whether you leave the key held down. If you do, Windows accepts multiple versions of the key until you release it.

These are useful techniques if, say, you're using the arrow keys to navigate a document or the Backspace key to delete a number of characters. They're decidedly *not* useful if you have mobility challenges that cause you to frequently bounce your finger on a key or hold down a key that you meant to press only once.

If you tend to press keys multiple times or hold keys down too long, the Filter Keys feature lets you filter out the extra characters that appear in these situations. To use this feature, first follow these steps to activate it:

1. Select **Start**, **All Programs**, **Accessories**, **Ease of Access**, **Change how your keyboard works**.

2. Activate the **Turn on Filter Keys** check box, as shown in Figure 9.9.

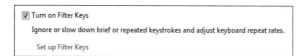

Figure 9.9: Activate Filter Keys to filter out unwanted keystrokes.

3. Click **Apply**. Don't click OK here because you'll need this window onscreen for the next two sections.

In Windows Vista, you can follow these same steps to turn on Filter Keys. In Windows XP, select **Start, Control Panel, Accessibility Options, Accessibility Options,** click the **Keyboard** tab, activate the **Use FilterKeys** check box, and then click **OK**.

With Filter Keys turned off, you next have to decide whether you never want multiple keystrokes or whether you want to control when multiple keystrokes are accepted by Windows.

Ignore Multiple Keystrokes

If your mobility issues mean that you tend to bounce your finger on the keys or hold down a key unintentionally, then your best bet is to tell Windows to ignore all the extra keystrokes that it would normally accept in these situations. Here's how:

1. Follow the steps in the previous section to activate Filter Keys, then click the **Set up Filter Keys** link.

2. Select the **Turn on Bounce Keys** option, as shown in Figure 9.10.

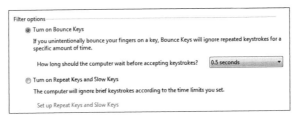

Figure 9.10: Activate Bounce Keys to tell Windows not accept multiple keystrokes.

3. Use the **How long should the computer wait before accepting keystrokes** list to select a time interval. If you press a key once and then press it again before this interval elapses (for example, if you accidentally bounce your finger on a key), Windows will

accept the first keystroke but ignore the second one. If you press the same key again after this interval elapses, Windows will accept that keystroke.

4. Click **OK**.

Control Multiple Keystrokes

On the other hand, you may occasionally want to hold down a key and have Windows accept multiple keystrokes. If you find that the default half-second delay is too short for your mobility needs, you can control that. Here's what you do:

1. Follow the steps in the earlier "Avoid Unwanted Keystrokes" section to activate Filter Keys, then click the **Set up Filter Keys** link.

2. Select the **Turn on Repeat Keys and Slow Keys** option.

3. Click the **Set up Repeat Keys and Slow Keys** link to display the window shown in Figure 9.11.

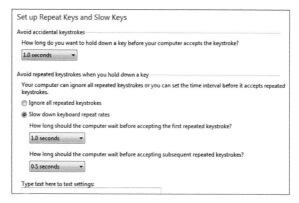

Figure 9.11: Use this window to configure when and how Windows accepts multiple keystrokes.

4. Use the **How long do you want to hold down a key before your computer accepts the keystroke** list to select a time interval. If you hold down a key for less than this time, Windows will not accept the keystroke.

5. Select the **Slow down keyboard repeat rates** option.

6. Use the two lists to set how long Windows waits before accepting the first repeated keystroke and the subsequent repeated keystrokes. If you tend to leave a key held down accidentally, increasing these times will help you avoid unwanted keystrokes.

7. Click **OK**.

Keeping Notifications Onscreen Longer

As you work with your computer, every now and then Windows or one of your applications will pester you by displaying a message in the notification area. For example, you see the message shown in Figure 9.12 whenever Windows has new updates that it wants you to install.

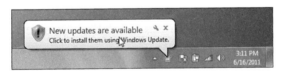

Figure 9.12: A notification from the aptly named notification area.

Notifications are useful because they keep you informed about what's happening on your computer, and they give you a quick way to do something about the notification message. For example, when you see the message shown in Figure 9.12, you click the message to see a list of updates available for your computer, and you can then install those updates with a click.

The rub is that the notification message stays onscreen for only about five seconds, which doesn't give you much time to read the message, decide whether you need to click it, and then perform the actual click. If you're too late, the message disappears—and you either have to wait for it to return (which might happen the next time you start your computer) or figure out some other way to perform whatever action the message requires.

One trick you can use is to move the mouse pointer over the notification. This action tells Windows to leave the message on the screen indefinitely, which then gives you time to contemplate the message at your leisure.

However, all of this assumes that you can manipulate your mouse fast enough to either click the notification or move the mouse pointer over it. If you find that you have trouble doing this, you can tell Windows to leave notifications onscreen for a longer time—up to five minutes, in fact. Follow these steps:

1. Select **Start**, **All Programs**, **Accessories**, **Ease of Access**, **Ease of Access Center**. You can also press **Windows logo key+U**.

2. Click **Make it easier to focus on tasks**.

3. Use the **How long should Windows notification dialog boxes stay open** list (see Figure 9.13) to select a time that makes sense for you.

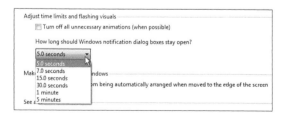

Figure 9.13: Use this list to tell Windows how long you want notifications to stay onscreen.

4. Click **OK**.

If you use Windows Vista, follow these same steps to set the notification time.

> **By the Way**
> If you use Windows XP, then I'm sorry to report that it doesn't have an equivalent setting.

Controlling Your Computer with Voice Commands

If you find that using a mouse and keyboard is too time-consuming, too difficult, or too frustrating, you may think you're out of luck—because how else are you supposed to control your computer? Fortunately, there *is* another way: voice commands. Using the Speech Recognition feature, you can speak commands into a microphone, and Windows will do your bidding.

Does it really work? Actually, most of the time, yes—it really does. Windows 7 has very good voice-recognition technology, and as long as you're in a relatively quiet room and speak clearly, Windows will recognize actions such as *click*, *double-click*, and *select*; commands such as *Save*, *Copy*, and *Close*; keystrokes such as *Backspace*, *Delete*, and *Enter*; and screen features such as *Minimize*, *Scroll*, and *Back*.

> **Good to Know!**
> One of Speech Recognition's handiest tricks is to say *Show numbers,* which then overlays a number over everything in the current window that can be clicked. You can then say the number of the item you want and say *OK,* and Speech Recognition will "click" that item for you *and* tell you the correct command name.

To get started, you need to attach a microphone to your computer. A microphone that's part of a headset is easiest to use, but you can also use a standalone microphone that sits on your desk.

With your microphone attached to your computer, your next task is to configure the Speech Recognition feature:

1. Select **Start**, **All Programs**, **Accessories**, **Ease of Access**, **Windows Speech Recognition**. The Speech Recognition window appears.

2. Click **Start Speech Recognition**. The Set up Speech Recognition Wizard appears and gives you an overview of the feature.

3. Click **Next**. The wizard asks what type of microphone you have.

4. Make your selection (such as Headset Microphone or Desktop Microphone), then click **Next**. The wizard displays a screen that tells you about the proper placement of your microphone.

5. After you've read the text and made the necessary adjustments, click **Next**. The wizard now displays some text for you to read aloud. (If anyone is nearby, you may want to give him or her a heads up about what you're up to.)

6. Read the text in your normal voice, then click **Next**. Now, the wizard asks whether it can examine your documents to look for words that it should learn.

7. This is a good idea, so select **Enable document review** and click **Next**. Now, the wizard wants to know how you want to activate speech recognition.

8. The easiest route here is to select **Use voice activation mode**, which means you can start Speech Recognition by saying "Start listening" and stop Speech Recognition by saying "Stop listening." Click **Next**. The wizard suggests that you print the Speech Reference Card, which contains a list of useful commands.

9. If you want to print the card, click **View Reference Card** and then click the **Print** button in the Help window that appears.

10. Return to the Set up Speech Recognition wizard (if you printed the card in the previous step), then click **Next**. The wizard wonders whether you want to start Speech Recognition automatically each time you start your computer.

11. This is a good way to go, so click **Next**. The wizard now offers to take you through a Speech Recognition tutorial, which enables you to practice the voice commands.

12. The tutorial is definitely worthwhile, so click **Start Tutorial**.

13. When you're done, click **Finish**.

Windows Vista uses essentially the same Speech Recognition program, so the steps I outlined here will work fine if you're a Vista user.

By the Way

Sadly, Windows XP doesn't come with its own speech-recognition feature.

With all that out of the way, you can start using Speech Recognition, which appears as a small window at the top of the desktop. You speak your commands, and Speech Recognition will either carry them out or will say, "What was that?" if it doesn't recognize what you said. In Figure 9.14, I've just said "Start menu," and not only has Speech

Recognition opened the Start menu but it has also echoed the command in its window.

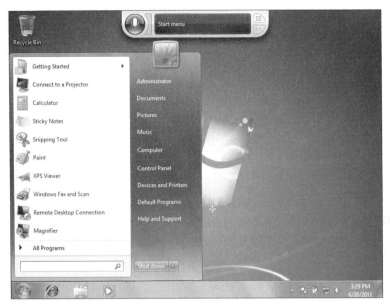

Figure 9.14: Speech Recognition at work: say "Start menu" to open the Start menu.

The Least You Need to Know

- If you have trouble manipulating the mouse, turn on the Mouse Keys feature to control the pointer from the keyboard.
- You can also activate the ClickLock feature to avoid having to hold down a mouse button while you drag things.
- You can also configure your computer to switch to a window by hovering over it with the mouse, and you can prevent windows from getting automatically arranged at the edges of the screen.

- For an easier time with the keyboard, you can turn on Sticky Keys, which enables you to press modifier keys one at a time.
- To avoid unwanted keystrokes, turn on Filter Keys. You can then turn on Bounce Keys to ignore multiple keystrokes or Slow Keys to control when Windows accepts multiple keystrokes.
- To bypass the mouse and keyboard altogether, activate and configure Speech Recognition, which enables you to run commands, enter keystrokes, and perform actions using your voice only.

Using Your Computer to Go Online

Part 3

There are all kinds of rhymes and reasons why the internet is, well, *everywhere* these days, but here's the main one: it's *useful*. Why phone or write to a company for a brochure when you can go to its website and see it (and more) right away? Why send a letter to someone that takes a few days to get there when you can send an email that arrives in a few minutes? Why root around dusty library stacks for hours to do your research when you can search any of the web's billions (yes, that right, *billions*) of websites from the comfort of your home? If you answered, "Beats the heck outta me" to any of these questions, then it's time to get you online—which is what happens in Part 3.

Setting Up a Network and Internet Access

Chapter 10

In This Chapter

- Figuring out internet service providers
- Setting up the equipment
- Getting yourself on the internet
- Disconnecting from the internet
- Treating yourself to wireless internet access

I wrote my very first Windows book way back in 1992. You can scour that book with a fine-toothed comb but won't find the word "internet" anywhere. Those were the good-ol' days when your social standing didn't depend on having both an email address and a web page, when "http://" was just a meaningless collection of letters and symbols to most people, and Bill Gates's billions could be counted using just your fingers.

Now, the internet's tentacles have insinuated themselves into every nook and cranny of modern life. Businesses from corner-hugging mom-and-pop shops to continent-straddling corporations are online, web pages are now counted in the tens of billions, and people send far more email messages than postal messages.

It truly is a wired world, as no doubt your kids and grandkids have been telling you—so if you feel like you're the only person left who isn't online, this chapter will help. I'll tell you exactly what you need to make it happen, and then I'll take you through the connection process.

Researching Internet Service Providers

If you have a hankering for, say, a cubic zirconia bangle bracelet or a Three Stooges bean bag set, all you have to do is call the Home Shopping Network and lay down your plastic.

> **What Can Go Wrong?**
>
> The internet is a place to have fun, learn new things, and connect with family and friends. However, I'd be remiss in my duties as your guide to this new world if I didn't caution you that the internet also has its share of nogoodniks that you need to avoid. Therefore, once you're online, be sure to also read the chapters in Part 4.

If you have a hankering to see some information about cubic zirconia bangle bracelets or Three Stooges bean bag sets, however, things aren't quite so easy. That's because the route to the internet isn't a direct one. Instead, you can only get there by engaging the services of a middleman—or, more accurately, a middle company: an *internet service provider* (*ISP* for short).

> **Definition**
>
> An **internet service provider (ISP)** takes your money in exchange for providing an internet account, which you need to get online.

An ISP is a business that has negotiated a deal with the local telephone company or some other behemoth organization to get a direct connection to the internet's highways and byways. These kinds of connections cost thousands of dollars a month, so they're out of reach for all but the most well-heeled tycoons. The ISP affords it by signing up subscribers and offering them a piece of the ISP's internet connection. After you have an account with an ISP, the connection process works as follows:

1. You use your modem to connect to the ISP.

2. The ISP's computer verifies that you're one of their subscribers.

3. The ISP's computer sets up a connection between your computer and the internet.

So before you can do anything on the internet, you have to set up an account with an ISP and then give Windows the details. Before we get to that, let's take a second to run through a few pointers when deciding which ISP to use.

Good to Know!

If the idea of setting up your own internet connection seems daunting, look for an ISP that will perform the installation and internet setup for you. Remember, too, that there's no shame in calling up a tech-savvy friend or family member to help you create the connection.

First, decide what type of connection you want, which will affect the kinds of ISPs you check out. There are two basic connection types:

- **Dial-up.** This type of connection uses your computer's modem to dial a phone number that connects the modem to an ISP's system. In general, dial-up connections are inexpensive but slow.

- **Broadband.** This type of connection uses a special external modem to connect to the ISP. Broadband connections are usually a bit more expensive than dial-up, but they are many times faster. Most folks use broadband these days.

The next couple sections take you through some specific ISP pointers for each type of connection, but here are four general tips to bear in mind when you're ISP shopping:

- Connection speeds are measured in either thousands of bits per second—usually abbreviated as kbps—or millions of bits per second—usually abbreviated as mbps. (A *bit* is the fundamental unit of information that computers deal with. For example, it takes eight bits to define a single character, such as "a" or even "ä.")

- Make sure the ISP offers a local or toll-free number for technical support.

- Deal with only large ISPs. There are still plenty of fly-by-night operations out there, and they're just not worth the hassle of dropped connections, busy signals, lack of support, or going belly-up when you most need them.

- If you can't decide between two or more ISPs, see what extra goodies they offer: space for your own content, extra email accounts, internet software bundles, and so on.

By the Way

Most people find that they spend a ton of time on the internet for the first few months as they discover all the wonders and weirdness that's available. After they get used to everything, though, their connection time drops dramatically.

Do It with Dial-Up

Here are some things to mull over if you're thinking about a dial-up connection:

- Most ISPs charge a monthly fee, which typically ranges from $5 to $30. Decide in advance the maximum that you're willing to shell out each month.

- When comparing prices, remember that ISP plans usually trade off between price and the number of hours of connection time. For example, the lower the price, the fewer the hours you get.

- It's important to note that most plans charge you by the minute or hour if you exceed the number of hours the plan offers. These charges can be exorbitant (a buck or two an hour), so you don't want that. Therefore, give some thought to how much time you plan to spend online. That's hard to do at this stage, but you just need to ballpark it. If in doubt, get a plan with a large number of hours (say, 100 or 150). You can always scale it back later.

- Most major ISPs offer an "unlimited usage" plan. This means you can connect whenever you want for as long as you want, and you just pay a set fee per month (usually around $20). This is a good option to take for a few months until you figure out how often you use the internet.

- All modems made in the last few years support a faster connection speed called 56K (or sometimes V.90), which offers a maximum speed of 56 kbps. If you have such a modem (and if you're not certain, it's probably safe to assume that you do), make sure the ISP you choose also supports 56K (almost all of them do nowadays).

- Make sure the ISP offers a local access number to avoid long-distance charges. If that's not an option, make sure it offers access via a toll-free number. (Note: watch out for extra charges for the use of the toll-free line.) Even better, some nationwide ISPs offer local access in various cities. This is particularly useful if you do a lot of traveling.

By the Way

A dial-up connection to the internet is just like making any other phone call, which means that anyone trying to call *you* will get a busy signal.

Head Down the Broadband Highway

Most people use broadband now for a simple reason: it's *way* faster than dial-up. Depending on the connection speed, it can be anywhere from 4 or 5 times faster to 20, 30, or even *50* times faster. That's a lot. (Another broadband bonus: you don't tie up your phone line when you're connected.) Here are some things to put on your "Broadband Shopping Notes" list:

- Most ISPs charge a monthly fee, which typically ranges from $15 to $60.

- Broadband requires a different kind of modem, which you usually rent from the ISP. Make sure you find out what the rental fee will be.

- When comparing prices, remember that broadband ISP plans usually trade off between price and connection speed. For example, a cheap plan may get you a 256 kbps connection while a more expensive plan might max out at 20 mbps.

- When you look at the broadband speed, you'll almost always see two numbers—one higher than the other. The higher rate is the *download speed*, which is the rate at which stuff from the internet is sent to your computer; the lower rate is the *upload speed*, which is the rate at which you send stuff from your computer to the internet. Most internet connections spend way more time downloading than uploading, so the download speed is really the one to watch.

- It's important to note that most plans put a monthly limit on the amount of data you can send back and forth, or the *bandwidth*. If you exceed that amount, you get charged extra (be sure to find out how much!).

Connecting the Equipment

Once your internet account is set up, your next task is setting up the equipment you'll need to make the connection. The next two sections take you through the specifics.

Dial-Up Details

If you use a dial-up internet connection, your telephone and modem will probably share the same line. In this case, you don't have to switch the cable between the phone and the modem all the time. Instead, it's possible to get a permanent, no-hassle setup that'll make everyone happy. The secret is that all modems have two telephone cable jacks in the back:

- **Line jack.** This one is usually labeled "Line" or "Telco" or has a picture of a wall jack.
- **Telephone jack.** This one is usually labeled "Phone" or has a picture of a telephone.

Follow these directions to set things up:

1. Run a phone cable from the wall jack to the modem's line jack.
2. Run a second phone cable from the telephone to the modem's telephone jack.

This setup lets you use the phone whenever you need it. The signal goes right through the modem (when you're not using it, of course) and lets you use the modem whenever you need it.

Broadband Basics

A *broadband modem* is a high-speed modem used for ADSL (*Asymmetric Digital Subscriber Line*), cable, or satellite internet access. In almost all cases, the ISP provides you with a broadband modem that's compatible with its service. Getting the broadband modem connected is the first step in using the modem to get on the internet.

I should mention right off the bat that almost all broadband ISPs offer an installation option, which is often free of charge. If that's the case with your ISP, then you should definitely get them to install your broadband modem for you to ensure that everything is working properly.

If you're going the self-installation route, begin by connecting and plugging in the modem's power adapter. Make sure the modem is turned off. If the modem doesn't come with a power switch, unplug the power adapter for now.

Next, attach the cable that provides the ISP's internet connection. For example, if you have an ADSL broadband modem, run a phone line from the nearest wall jack to the appropriate port on the back of the modem—which is usually labeled ADSL or DSL, as shown in Figure 10.1.

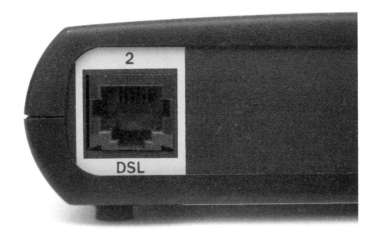

Figure 10.1: For an ADSL broadband modem, plug a phone cable into the DSL (or ADSL) port on the back of the modem.

Similarly, if you have a cable broadband modem, connect a TV cable to the cable connector on the back of the modem—which is usually labeled Cable, as shown in Figure 10.2.

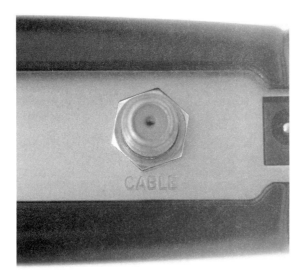

Figure 10.2: For a cable broadband modem, plug a TV cable into the cable connector on the back of the modem.

How you proceed from here depends on the ISP.

Finally, you need to connect the modem to your computer. Most broadband modems give you two ways to do this (see Figure 10.3):

- **Network** All broadband modems have a port on the back that's labeled Ethernet, LAN, or 10BASE-T. Run a network cable from this port to the network port on your computer (see Chapter 1 if you're not sure which port is the right one).

- **USB** Most newer broadband modems also come with a USB port on the back. If you're working with a computer that doesn't have a network port, you can use USB instead. Run a USB cable from the USB port on the modem to a free USB port on your computer.

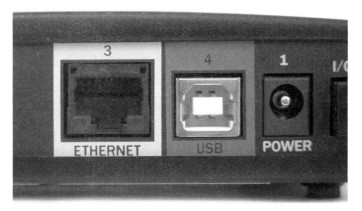

Figure 10.3: Almost all newer broadband modems come with both a network and USB port.

Turn on the broadband modem and wait until it makes a connection with the line. All broadband modems have an LED on the front that lights up to indicate a good connection. Look for an LED labeled Online, DSL, or something similar, and wait until you see a solid (that is, not blinking) light on that LED.

By the Way

Now, many ISPs insist that you register the broadband modem by accessing a page on the ISP's website and sometimes entering a code or the serial number of the modem. Read the instructions that come with your ISP's internet kit to determine whether you must first register your broadband modem online.

Setting Up the Connection

As you'll see in just a sec, you can build your internet connection with your bare hands—but you need to gather some raw materials first. Whether it's a dial-up or broadband connection to your internet account, you need to have the proper bits of information from your

ISP. In the bad old days (way back in the previous century), you needed reams of the most obscure and incomprehensible gobbledygook you had ever laid eyes on. Things are much more civilized nowadays, so you need to have just the following tidbits to *log on*:

- For a dial-up connection, you need the phone number you dial to connect to the ISP.
- For dial-up and broadband, you need the username (which may also be called your logon name) and password that you use to log on to the ISP.

Definition

To **log on** means to provide your ISP with your username and password to gain access to the internet.

With that information at your side, you're now ready to set up the account.

Create the Connection

Depending on who set up your computer, there's a chance your computer is already 'net-friendly. To find out, click the **Internet Explorer** icon in the taskbar (it's the fancy-looking "e" icon to the right of the Start button) to crank up the Internet Explorer Web browser. If a web page opens, then your internet connection is up and running. If you see the message, "Internet Explorer cannot display the webpage," you still have a few hoops that you need to jump through.

There's a good chance that your ISP sent you some kind of CD that contains the bits and pieces you need to get your connection running. If so, insert the CD and follow whatever instructions come your way to let the ISP handle all the hard stuff for you.

No CD? No problem. Whether your internet path is a dial-up road or a broadband highway, you start things off by following these steps:

1. Select **Start, Control Panel, Network and Internet, Network and Sharing Center** to open the Network and Sharing Center window.
2. Click **Set up a new connection or network**.
3. Click **Connect to the Internet**, then click **Next**. At long last, you see the two choices you've been waiting for: Broadband and Dial-up, as shown in Figure 10.4. (I talk about the third choice—Wireless—later in this chapter (see "Going Wireless").)

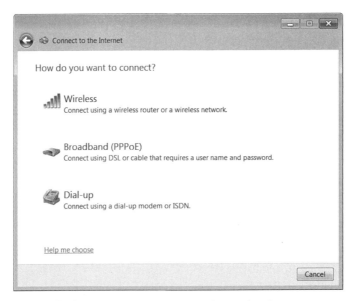

Figure 10.4: The inevitable fork in the internet road: select Broadband or Dial-up.

4. Click the connection type you want:

- **Dial-up.** If you click this type, you see a dialog box saying, "Type the information from your ISP." You use this dialog box to type in your ISP's phone number and your username and password. Figure 10.5 shows a completed version of this dialog box.

> **Good to Know!**
>
> For both dial-up and broadband connections, you can save yourself having to type your password every time you log on by activating the **Remember this password** check box.

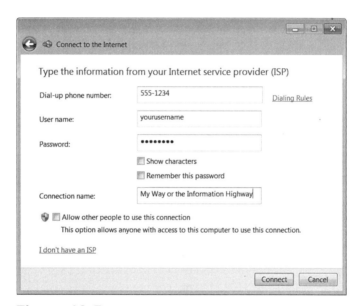

Figure 10.5: Use this dialog box to type in the information your ISP sent you.

- **Broadband.** If you click this type, you see a dialog box that's almost a carbon copy of the one in Figure 10.5. The only difference is that you don't have to type in the dial-up phone number.

5. Click **Connect**. Windows 7 creates the new connection and then takes it for a test drive.

If you're using Windows Vista, follow these same steps to get your connection up and running. To get an internet connection configured in Windows XP, select **Start**, **All Programs**, **Accessories**, **Communications**, **New Connection Wizard**.

If all goes well, you'd think there'd be music and fireworks—because hey, you're on the internet! But alas, no. You just get a rather ho-hum dialog box, shown in Figure 10.6. If you're not quite ready to do the internet thing yet, you should disconnect your dial-up connection—as described a bit later in the "Severing the Connection" section.

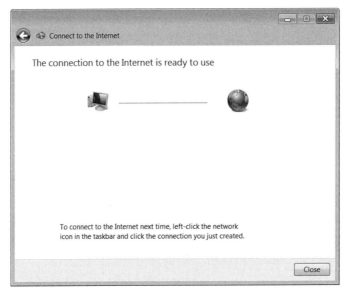

Figure 10.6: You see this dialog box if your internet connection was a success.

Future Connections

Windows 7 is considerate enough to establish a connection to the internet automatically after you set up your account. If you're using a broadband connection, then you'll probably want to keep it running full-time (for convenience). You can't do that with dial-up, so you need to disconnect after you're done and then reconnect later when you're looking for more internet action.

To reconnect to the internet, you have a couple choices:

- **Making the connection by hand:** click the **Network** icon in the taskbar's notification area (see Figure 10.7), click the internet connection you created, click **Connect**, and then click **Dial**.

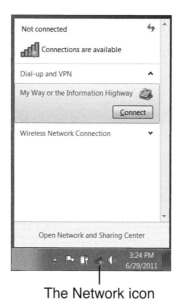

The Network icon

Figure 10.7: Click the **Network** icon, click your connection, and then click **Connect**.

- **Starting an internet program:** if you launch a program that requires an internet connection—such as Internet Explorer or Windows Live Mail—Windows 7 displays the Dial-up Connection dialog box shown in Figure 10.8. Click **Connect**, then click **Dial** to make things happen.

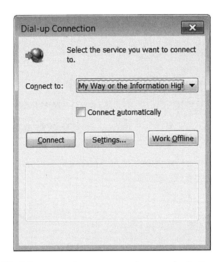

Figure 10.8: Now, when you launch internet-friendly programs such as Internet Explorer or Windows Live Mail, Windows 7 automatically prompts you to connect to the internet.

Good to Know!

For even faster service in the future, activate the **Connect automatically** check box. This command tells Windows 7 to bypass the Dial-up Connection dialog box and make the connection without pestering you.

Severing the Connection

When you've stood just about all you can take of the internet's wiles, you can log off by clicking the **Network** icon in the notification area, clicking your connection, and then clicking **Disconnect**, as shown in Figure 10.9.

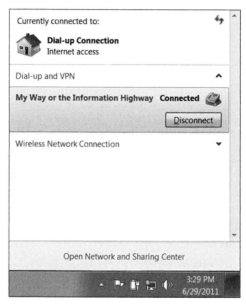

Figure 10.9: To disconnect, click the **Network** icon, click your connection, and then click **Disconnect**.

Going Wireless

Based on the internet connection you have so far, you may be wondering about a few things:

- If you have a second computer, is it possible for that computer to also use the internet connection?

- If your computer is a notebook or similarly portable PC, is it possible to lug the computer to some comfy spot—say, your favorite easy chair or your back patio—and still have access to the internet?

The answer to both questions is a resounding "Yes!" The key is a technology called *Wi-Fi* (it rhymes with *hi-fi*), which is short for wireless fidelity—although nobody ever uses the full phrase these days. The secret sauce is the "wireless" part of the name, which enables you to access your broadband internet connection without your computer being physically connected to the broadband modem.

Setting Up the Wireless Connection

That sounds like voodoo, I know, but it's the real deal. To set up a wireless connection, you need two things:

- Each computer that you want to go wireless must have a wireless network adapter. This component enables the computer to send and receive signals wirelessly. Almost all modern computers have this component built-in. How can you tell? Click the **Network** icon in the notification area. If you see **Wireless Network Connection**, as shown in Figure 10.10, then your computer is wireless-friendly. If not, then you need to purchase a wireless network adapter, which is usually a USB device that you plug into a free USB port on your PC.

- You need a device called a *wireless router*. This device (an example is shown in Figure 10.11) connects to your broadband modem, and it's through the wireless router that your computer connects to the internet.

Chapter 10: Setting Up a Network and Internet Access   213

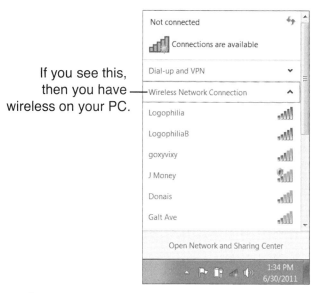

If you see this, then you have wireless on your PC.

Figure 10.10: If you see Wireless Network Connection when you click the Network icon, your computer is wireless-ready.

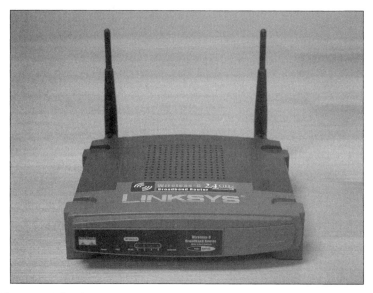

Figure 10.11: An example of a wireless router, with its telltale antennae (although most have a single antenna).

Once you have the wireless router, you need to connect it to your broadband modem. To do this, first turn off both the broadband modem and the router.

Examine the back of your wireless router and locate the port that it uses for the internet connection. Conveniently, some label this port "internet" (see Figure 10.12), whereas others use WAN or WLAN. Some annoying routers don't label the internet port at all but instead place the port off to the side so that it's clearly separate from the router's other ports. Run a network cable from the network port in the back of the modem (which, remember, is the one labeled Ethernet, LAN, or 10BASE-T) to the internet port in the back of the wireless router.

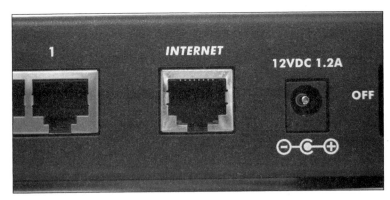

Figure 10.12: Run the network cable from the broadband modem to the internet (or WLAN) port in the back of the wireless router.

Configuring the Wireless Router

Your next step is to configure the wireless router for internet access. Unfortunately, there isn't a single, straightforward way to go about this. There are, in fact, *dozens* of possibilities—depending on the type of wireless router you have and the company you're using as your ISP. Obviously, I can't cover all of the possibilities here, but I'll be happy to give you the general steps. For the specifics, see the manual that came with the router and the instructions provided by your ISP.

The first thing you need to do is temporarily connect your computer to the wireless router. Run a network cable from the network port on your computer to a similar port on the back of the router (although not the internet or WLAN or WAN port used by the broadband modem).

Now, follow these steps to access the router's setup pages:

1. On the computer connected to the router, click the **Network** icon in the notification area, then click **Network and Sharing Center**.

2. Click **View full map**. Windows displays the Network Map window (see Figure 10.13), which contains a map of devices on your network. You should see an icon for the router. The name of the icon usually is the same as the router's model number. In Figure 10.13, for example, the router is the icon named D-Link DGL-4100.

What Can Go Wrong?

What happens if you don't see an icon for your wireless router? All is not lost, fortunately. Get out the router manual and dig through it until you find out the router's IP address, which will be something like 192.168.1.1. Start Internet Explorer, type that address in the Address bar, and press **Enter**.

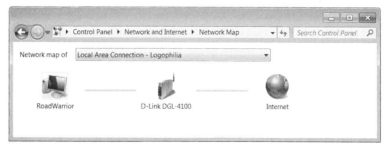

Figure 10.13: You should see an icon for your router in the Network Map window.

3. Click the router icon. The router prompts you to log on to the device.

4. Type the default username and password. (See the router manual for the logon details.)

5. Click **Log In** (or **OK**, or whatever). The router's setup pages appear.

Now that you're into the setup pages, you can make the necessary modifications. Using your router manual and ISP document as a guide, you should change the following things:

- **The type of internet connection.** This is usually either DHCP (if you have a broadband connection with a cable ISP) or PPPoE (if you have a broadband connection with an ADSL ISP). The latter also requires your connection's username and password.

- **The network name.** This is a name that you need to think of to uniquely identify your wireless network. This will make it easier for you to make the connection (as I describe in just a bit). The network name is often called the SSID.

- **The wireless security options.** To ensure that every nearby Tom, Dick, and Harry can't access your wireless network, you need to configure the security options. For the encryption type, choose WPA2—and then enter a password (which may be called, mysteriously, a "pre-shared key").

- **The administration password.** You use this password to access the router's setup pages. All routers come with a default password (usually *admin*), but you should change it so that other people can't access the setup pages.

When you've done all that, pat yourself on the back, save your changes, and then disconnect the network cable that's running from the computer to the router. (From now on, you can access the setup pages wirelessly if need be.)

Making the Wireless Connection

With your wireless router now hooked up to the broadband modem and configured with the internet connection type, the router will automatically create a connection to the internet. Your job now is to wirelessly tap into that connection:

1. Click the **Network** icon in the notification area. Windows displays a list of nearby wireless networks.

2. Click your wireless network. That is, click the network name that you provided in the previous section.

3. Click **Connect**. Windows prompts you to enter your wireless network password (which it calls a "security key").

4. Type the password, then click **OK**. Windows connects your wireless network, and you're free to surf the web wirelessly.

The Least You Need to Know

- If you'll be setting up your connection by hand, your ISP should provide you with the settings and data you need: the access phone number (for dial-up) and your username and password.
- To have both your phone and your modem available for use, run a phone cable from the wall jack to the modem's line port, and run a second cable from the phone to the modem's telephone jack.

- Making the leap to the internet is as easy as clicking the **Network** icon in the taskbar's notification area, clicking your connection, and then clicking **Connect**.
- To disconnect from the internet, click the Network icon in the notification area, click your connection, and then click **Disconnect**.
- To make a wireless connection to the internet, you need a Wi-Fi network adapter in your computer, and you need a wireless router connected to your broadband modem.

Surfing the Web

Chapter 11

In This Chapter

- Getting acquainted with the Internet Explorer window
- How to navigate from one web page to another
- Searching the internet for the information you want
- Using the World Wide Web to perform basic tasks

What is the World Wide Web? Well, I could sit here and tell you, as does the American Heritage Dictionary of the English Language, that it's "an information server on the internet composed of interconnected sites and files, accessible with a browser." I *could* do that, but I'm afraid your initial impression of the World Wide Web would be that it's excruciatingly *boring*. And if the web is anything, it's not boring. It's fascinating, frustrating, informative, infuriating, colossal, and corny, but dull? Never.

So, again, what is the World Wide Web? For starters, only pedants with overly pursed lips and fussbudgets with overly starched collars call it "the World Wide Web." The rest of us prefer just "the web," which is the less tongue-twisting short form that I'll use throughout this chapter. The web (ah, that's better) is a vast collection of documents called *pages*. How vast? Oh, there are now tens of *billions* of pages (give or take a few million). So you can imagine that these pages cover just about every topic under the sun (and few over the sun, to boot). You'll find everything from humble personal pages to humungous corporate sites; what-I-did-on-my-summer-vacation essays to all-the-news-that's-fit-to-print papers; full-blown biographies of the singer Nat King Cole to in-depth histories of the nursery rhyme Old King Cole.

The web may sound like just some giant encyclopedia, but it boasts something that you won't find in any encyclopedia printed on mere paper: interaction. For example, almost every web page in existence comes equipped with a few *links*. These are special sections of the document that, when clicked, immediately whisk you away to some other page on the site or even to a page on another site (which may be on the other side of town or on the other side of the planet). You can also use the web to play games, post messages, buy things, sell things, grab files and programs, and much more.

Your chariot for these internet adventures is a program called a web browser. In Windows, the chariot-of-choice is called Internet Explorer, and it's the subject of this chapter. You learn the nuts and bolts of the Internet Explorer window, how to use Internet Explorer to navigate web pages, and how to wield some Internet Explorer tools designed to make your web wandering easier.

Taking a Look at Internet Explorer

Assuming your internet connection is up and running, the most straightforward way to get Internet Explorer surfing is to click the **Internet Explorer** icon in the taskbar (it's the fancy-looking "e" to the right of the Start button). If you don't see that icon for some reason, you can also select **Start**, **All Programs**, **Internet Explorer**.

The first time you launch Internet Explorer, you may have to wrestle with the Set Up Windows Internet Explorer 8 Wizard. You can click the **Ask me later** button if you really don't feel like dealing with a wizard right now, but it'll just keep coming back (believe me). So it's better to get the entire setup rigmarole over with now. Here's what happens:

1. In the initial wizard dialog box, click **Next**. The Turn on Suggested Sites dialog box appears. Suggested Sites is an Internet Explorer 8 feature that displays a list of websites that are similar to whatever website you're currently viewing.

2. If Suggested Sites sounds like a good idea (you'll probably find it at least occasionally useful), select the **Yes, turn on Suggested Sites** option, then click **Next**. The Choose your settings dialog box appears.

3. Select the **Use express settings** option (it's much faster than configuring everything by hand), then click **Finish**. Internet Explorer displays the Welcome to Internet Explorer page, which is seriously uninteresting.

4. Press **Ctrl+W** to close the page.

That's it. Now it's on with the web show.

There's a good chance that you'll arrive at the MSN.com website, shown in Figure 11.1. (You may end up at a different site if your version of Windows 7 comes with custom internet settings.) Note that this screen changes constantly, so don't worry if the one you see looks different than the one shown in Figure 11.1.

MSN.com is Microsoft's internet starting point. (This kind of site is known as a *portal* in the web trade.) With its colorful layout, generous graphics, and loads of links, MSN.com is a typical example of the professionally designed pages that the big-time sites offer.

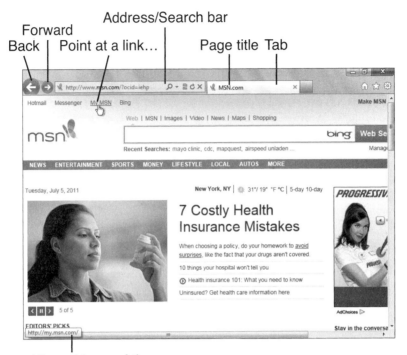

Figure 11.1: When you launch Internet Explorer, you usually end up at the MSN.com website.

 Good to Know!

If you don't like MSN.com (or whatever you have as Internet Explorer's default start page), it's easy to change it. First, surf to the page that you want to use as the new start page. Then select the **Tools, Internet Options** command to open the Internet Options dialog box. In the General tab, click **Use current**, and then click **OK**.

Before I show you how to use this page to see more of the web, let's take a minute or two and get our bearings by checking out the main features of the Internet Explorer window (most of which I've pointed out in Figure 11.1):

- **Page title.** The title of the current web page appears in a tab. See "Surfing with Tabs" later in this chapter to learn more.

- **Address/Search bar.** This area shows you the address of the current page. Web page addresses are strange beasts indeed. I'll help you figure them out in the following section. You also use this text box to search for websites (as explained ever so carefully in "Searching for Information on the Web" later in this chapter).

> **What Can Go Wrong?**
>
> When you surf to another page, Internet Explorer may pause for a while and then display a message that says: **This page cannot be displayed**. This often means that the website is kaput or down temporarily. However, I've found that Internet Explorer displays this message for no good reason a lot of the time, and pressing **F5** to refresh the page will bring the program to its senses.

- **Back** and **Forward.** You use these buttons to return to sites you've visited, as I explain in detail in the next section.

- **Content area.** This area below the tab takes up the bulk of the Internet Explorer screen. It's where the body of each web page is displayed. You can use the vertical scrollbar to see more of the current page.

- **Links.** The content area for most web pages also boasts a link or two (or ten). These links come in two flavors: images and text (the latter are usually underlined or in a different color than the rest of the text). When you place the mouse pointer over a link, Internet Explorer does two things (see Figure 11.1): changes the pointer into a hand with a pointing finger and displays, at the bottom of the window, the address of the linked page.

Web Page Navigation Basics

With that introduction out of the way, it's time to start wandering the web. This section runs through a few techniques for getting from one page to another. The most straightforward method is to click any link that strikes your fancy. Click the link, and you're immediately (depending on the speed of your internet connection) whisked to the other page. However, I suspect you may have a question or two at this point, so let's see if I can provide the answers.

How can I tell what's a link and what isn't?

That, unfortunately, is not as easy as it used to be. Originally, link text appeared underlined and in a different color. That's still the usual case for a link these days, but you can also get nonunderlined links as well as images that are links. The only real way to be sure is to move your mouse pointer over some likely looking text or an image and then watch what happens to the pointer. If it changes into the hand with a pointing finger (see Figure 11.1), then you know for sure that you have a link.

What if I know the address of the page I want to peruse?

Easy money. Here's what you do:

- Click inside the Address/Search bar, delete the existing address, type in the address you want to check out, and press **Enter**.
- If the address is one that you've visited recently, it should appear in the Address/Search bar's drop-down list. Click it in the list or press the **Down arrow** key to select it, then press **Enter**.

Why the heck are web addresses so, well, weird?

Probably because they were created by geeks who never imagined they'd be used by normal people. Still, they're not so bad after you figure out what's going on. Here's a summary of the various bits and pieces of a typical web address (or *URL*, which is short for Uniform Resource Locator, another geekism):

http://www.mcfedries.com/UsingComputerSeniors/index.asp

http://	This combination of letters and symbols tells the browser that you're entering a web address. Note that the browser assumes every address is a web address, so you don't need to include this part if you don't want to.
www.mcfedries.com	This is what's known as the domain name of the server computer that hosts the web page.
/UsingComputerSeniors/	This is the web server directory in which the web page makes its home. Web directories are similar to the folders you have on your hard drive.
index.asp	This is the web page's filename.

Is there any easier way to get somewhere?

If you're not sure where you want to go, the default start page (MSN.com) offers lots of choices. For example, click any of the categories near the top (News, Entertainment, Sports, and so on) to see links related to that topic.

By the Way

The domain name suffix most often used is .com (commercial), but other common suffixes include .gov (government), .org (nonprofit organization), .edu (education), and country domains such as .ca (Canada) and .uk (United Kingdom).

What if I jump to one page and then decide I want to double back to where I was?

You'll often find that you need to go back several pages and then leap forward again. Fortunately, Internet Explorer makes this easy, thanks to its Back and Forward toolbar buttons (which I helpfully pointed out back in Figure 11.1). Here's what you can do with them:

- Click **Back** to return to the previous page.
- Click **Forward** to move ahead to the next page.
- To jump directly to any page you've visited recently, click and hold the left mouse button on either the Back or Forward button to drop down a list of recent pages, then click the page you want.

Saving Your Favorite Sites

One of the most common experiences that folks new to web browsing go through is to stumble upon a really great site and then not be able to find it again later. They try to retrace their steps but usually just end up clicking links furiously and winding up in strange 'Net neighborhoods.

If this has happened to you, the solution is to get Internet Explorer to do all the grunt work of remembering sites for you. This is the job of the Favorites feature, which holds "shortcuts" to web pages and even lets you organize those shortcuts into separate folders.

Here's how you tell Internet Explorer to remember a web page as a favorite:

1. Navigate to the page that has struck your fancy.
2. Click **Favorites** (the star icon shown in Figure 11.2), then select **Add to favorites** to display the Add a Favorite dialog box.

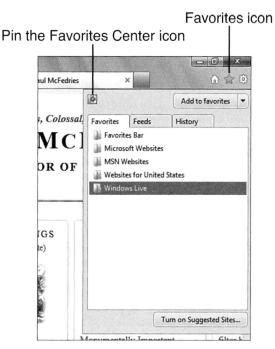

Figure 11.2: Click the **Favorites** icon to get things going.

> **Good to Know!**
>
> You can also display the Add a Favorite dialog box by pressing **Ctrl+D**.

3. The Name text box shows the name of the page, which is what you'll select from a menu later on when you want to view this page again. If you can think of a better name, don't hesitate to edit this text.

4. Click **Add** to finish.

After you have some pages lined up as favorites, you can return to any of them at any time by clicking the **Favorites** icon, clicking the **Favorites** tab, and then clicking the page title.

If you find yourself constantly reaching for the Favorites Center to get at your favorite pages, you might prefer to have the Favorites Center displayed full-time. You can do that by clicking the **Pin the Favorites Center** icon (see Figure 11.2). Internet Explorer then sets aside space on the left side of the window to display your Favorites list.

Surfing with Tabs

If you like, you can keep the current site in Internet Explorer and surf to a different site by pressing **Ctrl+N** to open a new Internet Explorer window. That's a neat trick, but it's not unusual to use it *too* often and end up with a half dozen or more Internet Explorer windows crowding your desktop. That's a lot of windows to wield. Fortunately, Internet Explorer comes with a nifty feature called *tabs* that lets you browse multiple sites in a *single* window. Nice!

The way it works is that you create a new tab in the current window, and you then use that tab to display a different web page. How do you create a new tab? Press **Ctrl+T** or click the **New Tab** button, pointed out in Figure 11.3. You then type the address you want and press **Enter** to load the page into the new tab.

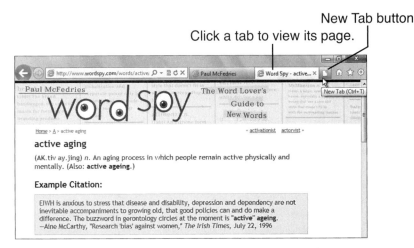

Figure 11.3: Internet Explorer lets you surf sites using tabs.

Here are a few tab techniques you can use to make surfing easier:

- If you see a link that you want to load into a separate tab, right-click the link and then select **Open in new tab**.
- To view a page that you have loaded in another tab, click the tab.
- To get rid of a tab, click it and then click the **X** that appears on the right side of the tab.

Downloading Files to Your Computer

As you click your way around the web, you find that some links don't take you to other pages but are instead tied directly to a file. In this case, Internet Explorer makes you jump through some or all of the following hoops:

1. In most cases, after you click the link to the file, you see a dialog box that asks whether you want to run or save the file. It's much safer to save the file, so click **Save** to tell Internet Explorer to store the file in your user account's Downloads folder.

2. If you elected to save the file, you'll eventually see the Download Complete dialog box, which offers three buttons:

    - **Open**. Click this button to launch the downloaded file.
    - **Open folder**. Click this button to open a window that displays the contents of the folder into which you saved the file. This is a good choice if you want to do something other than launch the file (such as rename it or sic your antivirus program on it).
    - **View downloads**. Click this button to display a list of all the files you've downloaded.

> **What Can Go Wrong?**
>
> Be careful about downloading files, because they can contain viruses that will wreck your system. To be safe, you should only download from reputable sites or from sites that you trust explicitly. If you plan on living dangerously and downloading files willy-nilly, at least get yourself a good antivirus program—such as McAfee (www.mcafee.com) or Norton (www.symantec.com)—and use it to check each file you download. See Chapter 15 for more information about staying safe on the web.

Searching for Information on the Web

Clicking around in the hope of finding something interesting can be fun if you have a few hours to kill. But if you need a specific tidbit of information *now*, then a click-click here and a click-click there just won't cut it. To save time, you need to knock the web down to a more manageable size, and Internet Explorer's Search feature can help you do just that.

The idea is straightforward: you supply a search "engine" (as they're called) with a word or two that describes the topic you want to find. The search engine then scours the web for pages that contain those words and presents you with a list of matches. Does it work? Well, it depends on which search engine you use. There are quite a few available, and some are better than others at certain kinds of searches. The biggest problem is that, depending on the topic you're looking for, the search engine may still return hundreds or even thousands of matching sites! You can usually get a more targeted search by adding more search terms and by avoiding common words. For example, suppose you want to know the airspeed velocity of an unladen swallow. If you search on just "swallow," you'll hit a wall of tens of millions of results. However, a search for "airspeed unladen swallow" will get you some pretty good results right off the bat.

A basic site search couldn't be easier: use the Address/Search text box to type the word or phrase you want to find, then press **Enter**. Internet Explorer passes the search buck over to the Bing search site, which then displays the results a few seconds later. As you can see in Figure 11.4, you get a series of links and descriptions. (Generally speaking, the higher the link is in the list, the more likely the page it points to matches your search text.) Clicking a link displays the page.

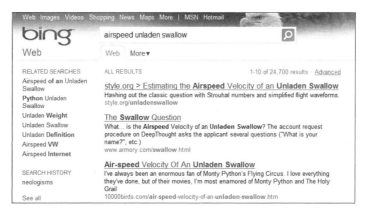

Figure 11.4: After the search is done, Internet Explorer displays a list of links to matching pages.

Internet Explorer uses Bing, which does a fine job of scouring the web—but you may want to try a few other search engines to see which one you like best. For example, pretty much the entire world uses Google (www.google.com), so you may want to try it and see what the fuss is about.

Some Tasks You Can Do on the Web

Now that you have a general idea of how to get around on the web and use Internet Explorer's basic features, it's time to put this web thingamajig to good use. To that end, the rest of this chapter takes you through a few useful tasks that you can perform without ever leaving your desk chair.

Share Photos

Throughout most of your life, you probably shared photos with family and friends by first taking your rolls of film to a photo-processing store, which then took a day or three to produce the prints that you'd then proudly pass around the room at your next family gathering or party.

Rolls of film have, of course, gone the way of the Victor-Victrola and the rotary-dial telephone. Photography is a resolutely all-digital world these days, so how does that affect how you share your photos? You actually have more choices than ever:

- You can still go to a photo-processing store, only now you take your camera's memory card instead of a roll of film.
- You can get yourself an inkjet printer and some photo paper to print your photos yourself.
- You can send a photo or two to someone you know via email, as I explain in Chapter 12.
- You can store your photos on the web for other people to see.

That last item may have caused you to raise an eyebrow. How on earth does one get photos on the web? And how are other people supposed to see those photos? The secret is the existence of various *photo-sharing sites*, which give you space for storing a bunch of photos as well as a unique address that you can give to other people to see those photos online.

Definition

A **photo-sharing site** is a website dedicated to storing digital photos and allowing other people to see those photos online.

Before I provide you with a list of photo-sharing sites to investigate, I should mention a few features to look for. The most important is storage space, because the more space you have, the more photos you can store. Most of the free sites offer between 100 MB and 1 GB of storage, which allows you to store between 20 and 200 photos. If you need more space, you can purchase it from the site. Also, look for sites that allow you to edit photos, turn your photos into calendars and greeting cards, and order prints.

Here are some photo-sharing sites to take a peek at (Figure 11.5 shows an example from the Picasa Web Albums site):

- **Flickr**   www.flickr.com
- **Picasa Web Albums**   picasaweb.google.com
- **Photobucket**   www.photobucket.com
- **Shutterfly**   www.shutterfly.com
- **Snapfish**   www.snapfish.com
- **Webshots**   www.webshots.com

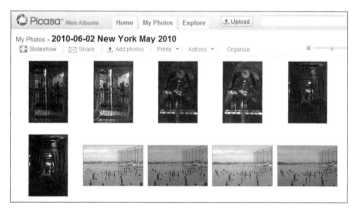

Figure 11.5: There are lots of photo-sharing sites on the web, including Picasa Web Albums.

I should mention here that Facebook is currently the web's most popular place to share photos. I didn't include it in the list because I'll be telling you all about it in Chapter 14.

View Maps and Get Directions

Can you get there from here? That's often a good question, and you're no doubt used to unfolding a paper map to find the answer. There's nothing wrong with that, but the web boasts a few *mapping sites* that enable you to view a map of just about any place on the globe. These sites enable you to zoom in to see details, zoom out for the big picture, and most importantly, they can give you street-by-street, turn-by-turn directions for getting from here to there.

Definition

A **mapping site** is a website that enables you to view and manipulate maps of streets and neighborhoods, towns and cities, states and regions, and countries and continents.

Here are four excellent mapping sites to try out:

- **Google Maps**   maps.google.com
- **MapQuest**   www.mapquest.com
- **Bing Maps**   www.bing.com/maps
- **Rand McNally**   maps.randmcnally.com

Of these, Google Maps is probably the most popular, so let's take it for a spin to see how you use it to get directions:

1. Use Internet Explorer to navigate to maps.google.com.
2. Type the name or address of the location you want to visit, then press **Enter**. Google Maps displays a map of the city or town, and it displays a "pin" at the location you specified.

3. Click **Get directions**. Google Maps asks you for the address of your starting point.

4. Type your starting address or location.

5. Click **Get Directions**. Google Maps displays the route on the map and also provides you with specific directions, as shown in Figure 11.6.

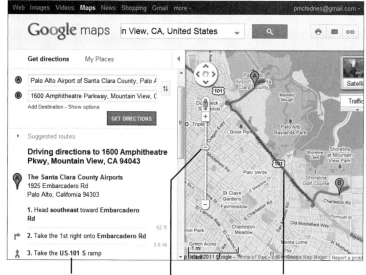

The directions appear here. | Your route appears on the map.
Drag the slider to zoom in and out of the map.

Figure 11.6: With Google Maps, you can get directions from point A to point B.

Read the News

If you're a news junkie, or if you just like to keep up with current events, then you're going to *love* the web. Not only do you get a wide variety of news stories from a similarly wide variety of news sources, but because websites are so easily and quickly updated, you can also be sure you're always seeing the latest news—not yesterday's news.

All that may explain why there's just so much news on the web. Chances are your favorite newspapers, magazines, and news shows have web-ified versions of themselves, so I suggest starting with those sites as a way of dipping your toe in the online news pool. (Run a search if you're not sure of the address of any of these sites.)

Once you have a handle on your favorite news sources, you can branch out a bit. There are four main categories of online news:

- **Newspapers and magazines.** It's a rare print news source that doesn't have an online equivalent these days, so you should be able to find just about any newspaper or magazine online. Examples include *The New York Times* (www.nytimes.com; see Figure 11.7), *The Washington Post* (www.washingtonpost.com), *Newsweek* (www.newsweek.com), and *The Economist* (www.economist.com).

> **By the Way**
>
> Most news sites offer at least some free articles and columns. Some sites (such as *The New York Times*) give you a maximum number of free articles per month (after which you must pay for a subscription to see more), while others charge a set fee for some articles.

- **TV news.** Any major network with a large news division will have a web version that offers extra content, such as videos and photos. Some sites to check out include CNN (cnn.com), Fox News (www.foxnews.com), ABC (abcnews.go.com), CBS (www.cbsnews.com), MSNBC (www.msnbc.msn.com), CBC in Canada (www.cbcnews.ca), and the BBC in Britain (news.bbc.co.uk).

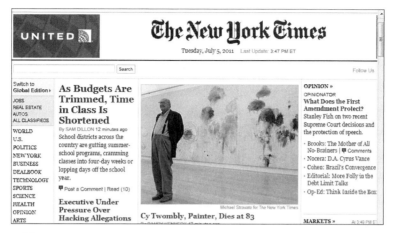

Figure 11.7: *The New York Times* offers a massive website with many news stories, investigative pieces, columns, and more.

- **Online news magazines.** Some web-based news sources exist as purely online magazines with no print equivalent. (Some in-the-know types call these *e-zines*.) Some of them are every bit as good as their offline counterparts and boast a variety of content, top-notch writing, and extras such as videos, photos, and podcasts (audio files that contain news stories or commentary). Take a gander at Slate (www.slate.com), Salon (www.salon.com), and Flak (www.flakmag.com).

- **News portals.** A *news portal* is a website that gathers news stories from hundreds of different online news sources. You can then search for stories or easily compare stories from multiple sources. The gold standard here is Google News (news.google.com), but also check out Bing News (www.bing.com/news) and NewsIsFree (www.newsisfree.com).

Research Your Family History

If you are trying to find your ancestors, the web boasts hundreds of genealogy sites. Either you can search directly using online resources such as birth and death records, or you can use dedicated (although not always free) genealogy sites such as the following (Figure 11.8 shows the popular Ancestry.com site):

- **Ancestry.com**   www.ancestry.com
- **Ancestor Hunt**   www.ancestorhunt.com
- **FamilyLink**   www.familylink.com
- **FamilySearch**   www.familysearch.org
- **Find a Grave**   www.findagrave.com
- **Genealogy**   www.genealogy.com
- **Geni**   www.geni.com
- **My Heritage**   www.myheritage.com
- **RootsWeb**   www.rootsweb.ancestry.com

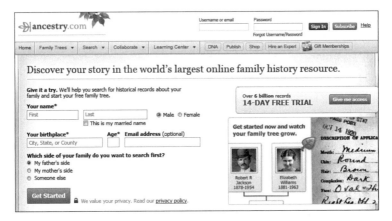

Figure 11.8: Ancestry.com is one of the most popular genealogy sites on the web.

Find Recipes and Cooking Tips

The web is home to a huge community of chefs of all levels operating in an amazing variety of styles and cuisines, and many of them are only too happy to share recipes and cooking advice. The easiest way to get started is to try a bit of what some people call *fridge Googling*. That is, you first check out what you have in your refrigerator, then use Google to run a search on those ingredients. Be sure to click **Recipes** on the left side of the results page to see only recipes. Also, you can use the check boxes in the **Ingredients** section to refine the search (see Figure 11.9).

Definition

Fridge Googling means running an internet search based on some or all of the contents of one's fridge, looking for a recipe based on those contents.

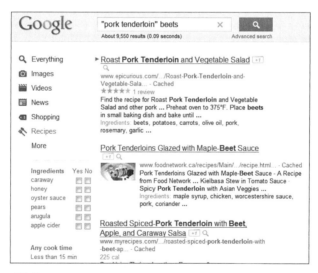

Figure 11.9: When you fridge Google, click **Recipes** and use the Ingredients check boxes to refine your search.

There are also tons of useful recipe sites on the web. Here's a taste:

- **AllRecipes**   www.allrecipes.com
- **Epicurious**   www.epicurious.com
- **CHOW**   www.chow.com
- **Cooking Light**   www.cookinglight.com
- **Food & Wine**   www.foodandwine.com
- **Food Network**   www.foodnetwork.com
- **iChef**   www.ichef.com
- **Simply Recipes**   www.simplyrecipes.com

Locate Health Information

Although the best source of health information is always your family doctor, that doesn't mean you shouldn't take advantage of the web to learn more about your health and any problems you may be experiencing.

For starters, here are some good general resources:

- **U.S. Department of Health and Human Services**   www.hhs.gov
- **Public Health Agency of Canada**   www.phac-aspc.gc.ca
- **National Institutes of Health**   www.nih.gov
- **Centers for Disease Control and Prevention**   www.cdc.gov
- **Veterans Health Administration**   www.va.gov/health

If you have a particular disease, illness, or health problem, do a search on "living with *condition*" (where *condition* is the name of the medical condition; for example, "living with diabetes," as shown in Figure 11.10).

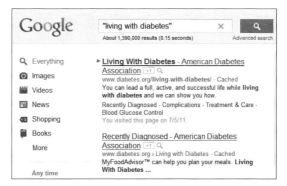

Figure 11.10: Run a web search on "living with *condition*."

The web is also home to websites for almost any major hospital or medical center (for example, the Mayo Clinic; see www.mayoclinic.com), organizations associated with a particular disease or condition (such as the American Cancer Society; see www.cancer.org), support groups (run a search on "*condition* support group"), famous doctors (such as Dr. Mehmet Oz; see www.doctoroz.com), and medical news (for example, Medical News Today; see www.medicalnewstoday.com).

The Least You Need to Know

- To start Internet Explorer, click the **Internet Explorer** icon in the taskbar. (Alternatively, select **Start**, **All Programs**, **Internet Explorer**.)
- To surf to another page, either click a link or type an address in the Address/Search bar and then press **Enter**. Use the toolbar's **Back** button to return to the previous page, and use the **Forward** button to head the other way.
- Click the **Favorites** button and then click the **Add to Favorites** command (or press **Ctrl+D**) to save a page to your Favorites list.

- Click the **Favorites** button to view your Favorites.
- To scour the web for a particular topic, type a word or two in the Address/Search box and press **Enter**.
- Besides being an excellent information resource, you can also use the web to share photos, get directions, read news, research your forebears, find recipes, and get health information.

Exchanging Email

Chapter
12

In This Chapter

- Giving Windows your email account particulars
- A look around Windows Live Mail
- How to compose and send an email message
- Attaching photos and other files
- How to receive and read incoming messages
- Using folders to organize your messages

The world passed a milestone of sorts a few years ago when it was reported that, in North America at least, more email messages are sent each day than postal messages. Now, email message volume is several times that of "snail mail" (as regular mail is derisively called by the wired set), and the number of e-notes shipped out each day is counted in the *billions.*

The really good news is that email has become extremely easy to use because email programs have improved over the years. As you see in this chapter, sending messages and reading incoming messages is a painless affair thanks to the admirable email capabilities of Windows Live Mail.

Getting Started with Windows Live Mail

As you might have guessed from the "Live" portion of its name, Windows Live Mail is part of Windows Live Essentials, which is the collection of those programs that Microsoft decided to leave out of Windows 7. To learn how to install it, review Chapter 3.

Once that's done, you fire up the program by selecting **Start**, **All Programs**, **Windows Live Mail**.

Setting Up Your Internet Email Account

Before Windows Live Mail loads for the first time, it calls in the Add an E-mail Account Wizard to handle the various steps required to divulge the details of the email account you have with your ISP (internet service provider). There are two possible routes here: the high (easy) road and the low (hard) road.

The High Road: Quick Account Setup

Windows Live Mail understands that many (perhaps even most) email accounts are really straightforward; with just a bit of information, it can glean the underlying details of the account. This process is relatively foolproof with well-known email providers such as Microsoft's Hotmail, and it seems to work okay with other companies, too.

In this scenario, all you need to know is your email address and your password. You enter that data in the Add an E-mail Account Wizard's initial dialog box, plus the display name you want to use (this is the name people see when you send them a message). Click **Next**, read the instructions (if any) that the wizard tells you to follow to complete the setup, and then click **Finish**.

The Low Road: Configuring an Account By Hand

If the wizard can't configure your email account automatically (if, for example, your email provider uses an oddball configuration, which isn't as uncommon as you might think), then you have to roll up your sleeves and do it yourself. Here's a rundown of the information you should have at your fingertips:

- Your email address

- The type of server the ISP uses for incoming email: *POP3*, *IMAP*, or *HTTP*

- The internet name used by the ISP's incoming *mail server* (a computer that your ISP uses to store and send your email messages); the mail server often takes the form mail.*provider*.com, where *provider* is the name of the ISP (note that your ISP might call this its *POP3 server*)

- The internet name used by the ISP's outgoing mail server (almost always the same as the incoming email server); some ISPs call this their *SMTP server*

- Whether your ISP's outgoing mail server requires authentication (most do nowadays)

- Whether your ISP requires you to use special port numbers (You can think of ports as communications channels, and Windows Live Mail and your ISP must be tuned in to the same channel for things to work. If you don't have any information on this, then your ISP probably uses the standard port numbers—so you don't have to sweat this part.)

- The username and password for your email account. (These are almost always the same as your internet logon name and password.)

> **Definition**
>
> The acronyms and abbreviations are thick on the ground in this section. You don't have to understand them to send and receive email, but here's what they mean just in case you're interested: **POP** stands for Post Office Protocol; **IMAP** stands for Internet Message Access Protocol; and **SMTP** stands for Simple Mail Transfer Protocol.

Here's what happens:

1. In the initial wizard dialog box, enter your address in the **E-mail address** text box and your password in the **Password** text box.

2. Use the **Display Name** text box to type the name you want other folks to see when you send them a message (most people just use their real name), then click **Next**.

3. Under the **Incoming server information** heading, use the **Server type** list to specify the type of email server your ISP uses; most are **POP**.

4. Use the **Server address** text box to enter the name of the server that your ISP uses for incoming mail. Also, change the **Port** value if your ISP uses a port other than the one shown.

5. Use the **Login user name** text box to enter your email username (this should already be filled in for you) or email address (whichever one you're supposed to use to log in).

6. Under the **Outgoing server information** heading, use the **Server address** text box to enter the name of the server that your ISP uses for outgoing mail. Also, change the **Port** value if your ISP uses a port other than the one shown.

7. Activate the **Requires authentication** check box if your ISP's outgoing mail server does the authentication thing. Figure 12.1 shows a sample dialog box filled in with the email details.

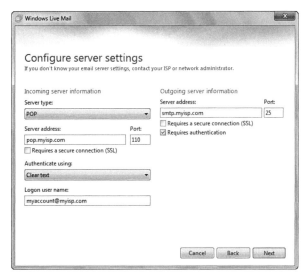

Figure 12.1: Use Windows Live Mail to ship and receive internet email messages.

8. Click **Next** to get your account set up.
9. Click **Finish**.

Touring Windows Live Mail

By default, Windows Live Mail is set up to go online and grab your waiting messages when you launch the program. We'll get there eventually, but for now, just close the Connect dialog box if it shows up.

At long last, the Windows Live Mail window shows itself, and it looks much like the one in Figure 12.2.

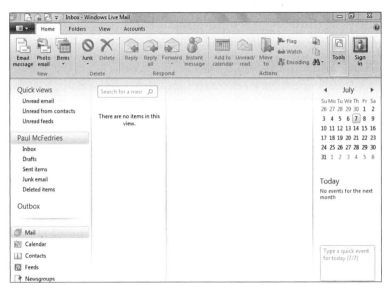

Figure 12.2: The Windows Live Mail window.

The Folder pane on the left lists the various storage areas that come with Windows Live Mail. I talk about folders in more detail later in this chapter. For now, here's a summary of what the default folders are all about:

- **Quick views**   This section offers special "views" of your messages, such as Unread email, which shows you all the messages that you haven't read yet.

- **Inbox**   This folder is where Windows Live Mail stores the email messages you receive.

- **Drafts**   This folder stores messages that you're in the middle of composing and have saved.

- **Sent items**   This folder stores a copy of the messages you've sent.

- **Junk email**   This folder is the Siberia to which Windows Live Mail exiles suspected spam messages. See Chapter 16 for more about dealing with spam.

- **Deleted items** This folder stores the messages that you delete.
- **Outbox** This folder stores messages you've composed but haven't sent yet.

Sending an Email Message

Let's begin the Windows Live Mail tour with a look at how to foist your e-prose on unsuspecting colleagues, friends, and family. This section shows you the basic technique to use, then gets a bit fancier in discussing the Contacts list, attachments, and other Windows Live Mail sending features.

Compose and Send a Message

Without further ado, here are the basic steps to follow for firing off an email message to some lucky recipient:

1. Select **Home**, **Email message** in the Windows Live Mail ribbon. (Or, if you're a keyboard fan, press **Ctrl+N**.) You end up with the New Message window on-screen, as shown in Figure 12.3.

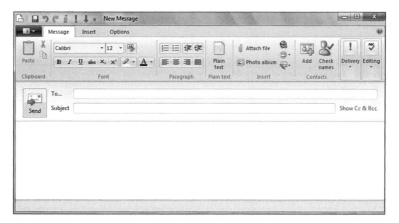

Figure 12.3: You cobble together an email message in the New Message window.

2. In the **To** text box, type the email address of the recipient. (It's perfectly acceptable to enter multiple addresses in this text box. Use a semicolon [;] or a comma [,] to separate each address.)

Good to Know!

The address you put in the To box is the "main" recipient of the message. However, it's common to send a copy of the message to a secondary recipient. To do that, click **Show Cc and Bcc** and then enter that recipient's email address in the **Cc** text box. (Again, you can enter multiple addresses if you're so inclined.) What about the Bcc text box? That's for a *blind courtesy copy,* which delivers a copy of the message to a specified recipient—but none of the other recipients see that person's address.

3. Use the Subject line to enter a subject for the message. (The subject acts as a title for your message. It's the first thing your recipient sees, so it should accurately reflect the content of your message, but it shouldn't be too long. Think *pithy.*)

4. Use the large, empty area below the Subject line to type the message text (also known as the *message body*). For the most part, you can just type your message as though you were typing a letter. One common mistake you should avoid is typing EVERYTHING IN CAPITAL LETTERS, WHICH MAKES IT LOOK AS THOUGH YOU'RE SHOUTING.

5. Use the buttons and other options in the **Message** tab to change the font, format paragraphs, and more.

6. When your message is fit for human consumption, click **Send** (or press **Alt+S**). Windows Live Mail sends the message—no questions asked.

After your message is sent, Windows Live Mail saves a copy of it in the Sent Items folder. This is handy because it gives you a record of all the missives you launch into cyberspace.

Use the Contacts List

If you find yourself with a bunch of recipients to whom you send stuff regularly (and it's a rare emailer who doesn't), you soon grow tired of typing their addresses by hand. The solution is to toss those regulars into the Contacts list. That way, you can fire them into the To or Cc lines with just a few mouse clicks.

Here's how you add someone to the Contacts list:

1. In Windows Live Mail, select **Home**, **Items**, **Contact**. (Keyboard diehards can press **Ctrl+Shift+C**.) Windows Live Mail conjures up the Add a Contact window, shown in Figure 12.4.

2. In the **Quick add** tab, enter the person's first and last names.

3. Use the **Personal email** text box to enter the recipient's address. Figure 12.4 shows an example window filled in.

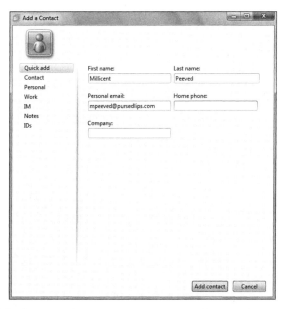

Figure 12.4: Use this window to spell out the particulars of the new recipient.

4. Fill in the person's phone number and company name (as well as the fields in the other tabs, if you feel like it).

5. When you're done, click **Add contact** to add the new recipient.

After you have some folks in your Contacts list, Windows Live Mail gives you a ton of ways to send them a message. Here's my favorite method:

1. In the New Message window, click **To**. Windows Live Mail displays the Send an E-mail dialog box.

2. Click the contact name.

3. Click **To** (or **Cc** or **Bcc**).

4. Repeat steps 2 and 3 to add more folks as needed for your message.

5. Click **OK**.

Email a Photo

Most of your email messages will be text-only creations. However, it's also possible to send entire files along for the ride. Such files are called, naturally enough, *attachments*. They're very common in the business world, and it's useful to know how they work.

Definition

An **attachment** is a separate file, such as a photo or text document, that accompanies an email message.

Probably the most common type of attachment you'll send is a photo, so let's start with that. Here's how you attach a photo to an email message:

1. In the New Message window, click inside the message body area, type the message you want to include (for example, a description of the photo), and press **Enter**.

2. Select **Insert, Single photo**. The Insert Picture dialog box appears.

3. Click the file you want to attach, then click **Open**. Windows Live Mail returns you to the New Message window, where you see the image in the message body (see Figure 12.5).

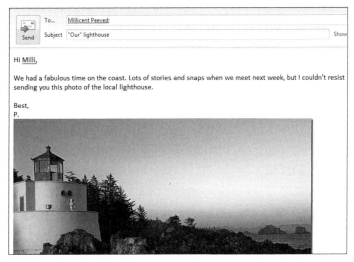

Figure 12.5: An email message with a photo shoehorned in the message body.

Email Other Types of Files

To send any other type of file, the steps are slightly different:

1. In the New Message window, compose your message.

2. Select **Insert, Attach file**. The Open dialog box appears.

3. Click the file you want to attach, then click **Open**. Windows Live Mail returns you to the New Message window, where you see the name of the file (and its size) below the Subject line (see Figure 12.6).

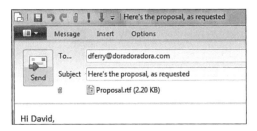

Figure 12.6: An email message with a file attached.

Getting and Reading Email Messages

Some people like to think of email as a return to the days of *belles-lettres* and *billets-doux* (these people tend to be a bit pretentious). Yes, it's true that email has people writing again, but this isn't like the letter writing of old. The major difference is that email's turnaround time is usually much quicker. Instead of waiting weeks or even months to receive a reply, a return email may take as little as a few minutes or hours.

So if you send a message with a question or comment, chances are you'll get a reply coming right back at you before too long. Any messages sent to your email address are stored in your account at your ISP. Your job is to use Windows Live Mail to access your account and grab any waiting messages. This section shows how to do that and what to do with those messages after they're safely stowed on your computer.

Get Your Messages

Here are the steps for getting your email messages:

1. Select **Home**, **Tools**, **Send/Receive** (or press **F5**).

2. Windows Live Mail connects to the internet (if necessary), accesses your mail account, absconds with any waiting messages, and then stuffs them into the Windows Live Mail Inbox folder. Disconnect from the internet if you no longer need the connection.

3. If it's not already displayed, click the **Inbox** folder so you can see what the e-postal carrier has delivered.

Note, too, that when you're working online, Windows Live Mail automatically checks for new messages every 10 minutes.

Read Your Messages

Figure 12.7 shows the Inbox folder with a few messages. The first thing to notice is that Windows Live Mail uses a bold font for all messages you haven't read yet. You also get information about each message in the middle column (including the message subject, who sent it, and when you received it). If you see a paper clip icon in this area (see Figure 12.7), it means the message is accompanied by a file attachment. See the next section, "Handle File Attachments."

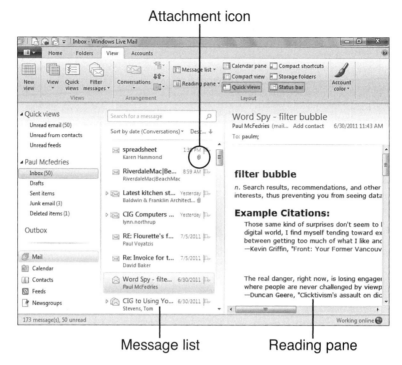

Figure 12.7: After you've pilfered your incoming messages from your ISP, they get stored in your Inbox folder.

Windows Live Mail offers two methods for seeing what a message has to say:

- Click the message in the Inbox folder. Windows Live Mail displays the text of the note in the reading pane. After a few seconds, Windows Live Mail removes the bold from the message to indicate that it has been read.

- Double-click the message in the Inbox folder. (For the heck of it, you also can press **Ctrl+O** or just **Enter**.) This method opens the message in its own window.

Handle File Attachments

As I mentioned earlier, if you get a message that has one or more files tied to it, you will see a paper clip icon within the message list. Windows Live Mail gives you a few ways to handle any attachments in the current message:

- **Saving the file** Select **File, Save, Save attachments** to open the Save Attachments dialog box. If there are multiple files, use the Attachments To Be Saved list to select the ones you want to save. Use the Save To text box to specify where you want the files to be stored (click **Browse** to choose the folder from a dialog box). Then, click **Save** to dump the file (or files) onto your hard disk.

- **Saving the file from the reading pane** Right-click the file in the upper-left corner of the reading pane, click **Save as**, and follow the steps I just took you through.

- **Opening the file** If you just want to see what's in the file, you can open it. To do that, right-click the file in the upper-left corner of the reading pane, then click **Open**.

> **What Can Go Wrong?**
>
> Although Windows Live Mail makes it easy to deal with attachments, you should never just blithely open an attached file because you may end up infecting your computer with a virus. To learn more about how to protect yourself from virus attachments, see Chapter 16.

Do Something with a Read Message

This section gives you a rundown of all the things you can do with a message after you've read it. In each case, you either need to have a message selected in the Inbox folder or have the message open. Here are some options:

- **Send a reply**   You can email a reply to the sender by selecting **Home**, **Reply**. (The keyboard route is **Ctrl+R**.)

- **Send a reply to every recipient**   If the note was sent to several people, you may prefer to send your response to everyone who received the original. To do that, select **Home**, **Reply all**. (The keyboard shortcut is **Ctrl+Shift+R**.)

- **Forward the message to someone else**   To have someone else take a gander at a message you received, you can forward it by Selecting **Home**, **Forward**. (Keyboard dudes and dudettes can press **Ctrl+F**.)

> **By the Way**
>
> A forwarded message contains the original message text, which is preceded by an "Original Message" heading and some of the message particulars (who sent it, when they sent it, and so on). If you want your recipient to see the message exactly as you received it, select **Home**, click the lower half of the **Forward** button, and then click **Forward As Attachment**.

- **Move the message to some other folder**   If you find your Inbox folder getting seriously overcrowded, you should think about moving some messages to other folders. The easiest way to do this is to drag the message from its current folder and drop it on the other folder in the Folders list. If that's too easy, select **Home**, **Move to** (or press **Ctrl+Shift+V**). In the Move dialog box that shows up, select the destination folder and then click **OK**.

- **Delete the message**   If you don't think you have cause to read a message again, you may as well delete it to keep the Inbox clutter to a minimum. To delete a message, select **Home**, **Delete**, or click the **Delete** button. (A message can also be vaporized by pressing **Ctrl+D** or by dragging it to the Deleted Items folder.) Note that Windows Live Mail doesn't get rid of a deleted message completely. Instead, it just stores it in the Deleted Items folder. If you later realize that you deleted the message accidentally (insert forehead slap here), you can head for the Deleted Items folder and move the message back to the Inbox.

Creating Folders to Store Your Messages

Right out of the box, Windows Live Mail comes with the seven prefab folders that I described earlier in this chapter. Surely that's enough folders for anyone, right?

Maybe not. Even if you're good at deleting the detritus from your Inbox folder, it still won't take long before it becomes bloated with messages and finding the note you need becomes a real needle-in-a-haystack exercise. What you really need is a way to organize your mail. For example, suppose you and your oldest granddaughter exchange a lot of email. Rather than storing all her messages in your Inbox folder, you could create a separate folder just for her messages. You could also create folders for each of your other grandkids, for the internet mailing lists you subscribe to, for current projects, or for each of your regular email correspondents. There are, in short, 1,001 uses for folders, and this section tells you how to create your own.

To create a new folder, follow these steps:

1. Select **Folders**, **New folder** to display the Create Folder dialog box.

2. In the **Select the folder** … list, highlight the folder within which you want the new folder to appear. For example, if you want your new folder to be inside your inbox, click the **Inbox** folder.

3. Use the **Folder name** text box to enter the name of the new folder.

4. Click **OK**.

The Least You Need to Know

- To start Windows Live Mail, select **Start**, **All Programs**, **Windows Live Mail**.
- To compose a message, select **Home**, **Email message**, type the address and a Subject line, fill in the message body, and then click **Send**.
- To send a photo, select **Home**, **Email message**, fill in the message particulars, and then select **Insert**, **Single photo**.
- To receive messages, select **Home**, **Tools**, **Send/Receive**.
- Make liberal use of folders to organize your messages. You create new folders by selecting **Folders**, **New folder**.

Chapter 13
Getting the Most from Online Shopping

In This Chapter

- The pros and cons of shopping in cyberspace
- Researching products, prices, and retailers online
- A buyer's guide to buying things online
- Booking your next vacation online
- Getting great deals with online coupons

There is, as you've probably discovered by now, a long list of things to do while you're online. You can read news, watch videos, and find information on just about any topic you can think of (and quite a few more that would never even cross your mind). However, there's a good chance that your list of online tasks doesn't include shopping. After all, buying stuff is something you do at the mall, at the corner store, or at some other locale made of bricks and mortar—where you can see and feel your purchases. Who'd want to spend money in the vaporous, neither-here-nor-there world of cyberspace?

You'd be surprised. Online shopping is a multi-billion-dollar deal these days. In fact, it's estimated that online shopping will blossom into a nearly $300-billion-a-year market by 2015. That's a lot of cash (or really, plastic), and it means that millions upon millions of would-be purchasers are researching and buying things while still in their pajamas.

This chapter introduces you to online shopping and takes you through the nuts and bolts of buying things online.

Online Shopping: The Pros and Cons

Shopping online in your pajamas is optional, fortunately, but the conveniences of buying online are not:

- You save time, gas, and—depending on the time of day and the destination—frustration by foregoing a trip to the mall. Plus, if you don't walk as well as you once did, shopping online saves a lot of legwork.

- Your selection is almost always much larger than it is in a physical store. That makes sense, because a real-world retail store only has so much space—whereas an online retail store probably has either a massive warehouse or can source goods from multiple vendors.

- You can easily comparison shop to get the best deal. Comparison shopping offline requires several trips to several stores in several malls, but online retailers are only a few clicks away.

Are there downsides to online shopping? Yes:

- The biggest drawback is almost certainly the fact that you can't touch, try on, or get a good look at the items you buy online. This is problematic for dresses and shoes, but it's not a big deal for books and electronics (assuming you know what you want).

- You have to watch out for exorbitant shipping fees and hidden service charges. I'll talk about how to avoid these charges a bit later in the chapter (see "Buying Things Online").

- You don't get the immediate satisfaction of an in-store purchase. Fortunately, it doesn't take forever to get your stuff when you shop online. Depending on the type of shipping you select and how far your purchase has to travel, you can usually get your goods in your mitts in as little as a day—but more likely two or three days.

> **What Can Go Wrong?**
>
> Sadly, whenever money's involved, criminals and scam artists are all too often lurking in the weeds. Online shopping is quite safe, but there are a few pitfalls to be wary of. For some pointers, see Chapters 15 and 17.

Doing Your Research

As I mentioned in the previous section, one of the chief advantages of shopping online is that you can use the web's abundant resources to do some research before you spend a dime. Not only can you research products to find the one that best suits your needs, but you can also do some comparison shopping to find the best price—and you can research online retailers to make sure you're purchasing from a reputable outfit.

And even if you have no intention of actually purchasing things online, you can at least use the web's research tools to make some decisions up front without running all over town. The next three sections provide the research details.

Products

Whether you're looking for a computer or a coffeemaker, a barbecue grill or a Barbie doll, it's a lead-pipe cinch that someone has reviewed it and posted that review online for all to read. I'm not talking here about little Johnny, the budding computer geek, proclaiming the latest Hewlett-Packard PC to be "Awesome!" on his blog (although, of course, there's no shortage of that kind of thing). Rather, I'm talking about in-depth, non-partisan reviews by professionals who really put products to the test and tell you the pros and cons of each piece of equipment.

> **Good to Know!**
>
> When you read a review, be sure to note the date it was published. If it was quite a while ago, the review may be talking about an older version of the product.

Product-review sites are a dime a dozen (if that), but a few are really good. Here are my recommendations:

- **Consumer Reports (www.consumerreports.org)** This is the web home of the famous magazine, and as you may expect, it's chock full of great information. You get buying guides (see Figure 13.1); reviews of specific products, ratings, and recommendations; and much more. Note, however, that some information is available only to subscribers.

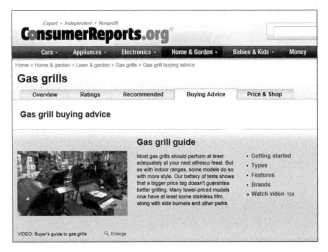

Figure 13.1: Consumer Reports is one of the best sites for product buying guides and reviews.

- **Consumer Search (www.consumersearch.com)** The tagline of this large, sprawling site is, "Love what you buy," and the site helps you do that by offering tons of reviews and recommendations for a huge variety of products.

- **CNET (http://reviews.cnet.com/)** This massive site has a Reviews section that covers tons of products. Each review is simply laid out with headings such as Pros, Cons, Suitability, Value, and Suggestions. The layout of the site leaves something to be desired, so use the search engine to find what you want.

- **Epinions (www.epinions.com/)** This massive (and massively popular) site is about reviews written by regular people who own the products they're talking about. You get the pros and cons, a review, and ratings for characteristics such as durability, style, and ease of cleaning.

- **Top Ten Reviews (www.toptenreviews.com)** As its name implies, this site lists the top ten products in each category and offers not only a review of each product but also an extensive list of features and tells you which products have them.

Besides these general review sites, there are also lots of review sites that are more targeted. For example, Amazon (www.amazon.com) has lots of book reviews, Edmunds (www.edmunds.com; see Figure 13.2) specializes in car reviews, and Good Housekeeping (www.goodhousekeeping.com) focuses on household products.

Good to Know!

Besides checking specific sites for reviews of a particular component, you can also try running a Google search that includes the product name and the word *review*. Be sure to search not only the web but also Google Groups (groups.google.com).

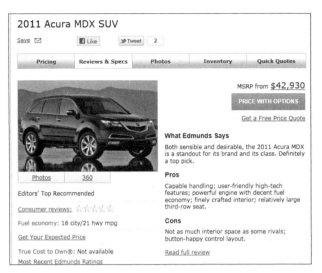

Figure 13.2: If you're in the market for a used or new car, Edmunds is a great place to start your research.

Prices

After you've read the reviews and know exactly what you want, your next step as a savvy shopper is to find the best price. You could do that by jumping around to various online retailers, searching for your product, and making note of the price each time. However, plenty of sites will do all the hard work for you. I'm talking about the web's price-comparison sites—sometimes called *shopping portals*—where you select or specify the product you want and the site returns the product listings from a number of online retailers. You can then compare prices with just a few mouse clicks.

Here are some decent shopping portals to check out:

- **Become (www.become.com)** This site shows you not only the prices for each listing but also the product's rating at each store (1 to 5 stars, based on user reviews).

- **CNET Shopper.com (http://shopper.cnet.com/)** This is the Shopper.com section of the CNET site. Its nicest feature is that for each store returned in the listings, you get the store's rating (1 to 5 stars) and whether the store currently has stock of the item—and if you enter your ZIP code, the taxes and shipping fees are displayed (see Figure 13.3).

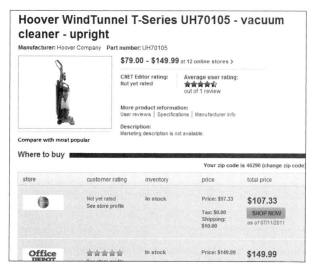

Figure 13.3: CNET's Shopper.com site not only compares prices but also provides each store's rating, stock, taxes, and shipping costs to your ZIP code.

- **Google Product Search (www.google.com/products/)** This site (formerly known as Froogle) applies the awesome power of Google's search engine to online products. You search on the name of the product you want, and Google returns product listings from around the web.

- **PriceGrabber.com (www.pricegrabber.com)** This is one of the most popular shopping portals, and no wonder—because, for each product, you get tons of information: price, stock, product details, user reviews and discussions, expert reviews, seller rating, and taxes and shipping for your ZIP code. What more could you want?

- **Shopzilla (www.shopzilla.com)**   This site doesn't have all the bells and whistles that you see with some of the other sites, but it often returns a broader array of listings and has all the basic information you need: price, taxes, shipping, product details, and product reviews.

- **Yahoo! Shopping (http://shopping.yahoo.com/)**   Lots of people like this section of Yahoo! because it provides all the standard shopping portal data and gives you full product specifications, user ratings, and the ability to send listings to a mobile phone (perfect if you're doing your shopping offline).

> **Good to Know!**
>
> If you're looking for a real bargain, shopping retail usually isn't the best way to go. This is particularly true online, where you have a number of other options. For example, check out the various online auction sites (especially eBay: www.ebay.com), where you can bid on used or new products and deals are often a click away. Also, be sure to check in with online classified sites (particularly Craigslist: www.craigslist.org).

Online Retailers

With hundreds of online retailers, how can you tell the e-commerce stars from the fly-by-night shysters? The best way is to ask your friends, family, and colleagues who they've used and had good experiences with in the past. Because these are people you trust, you can rely on the information you get.

Besides that, you can also go by the ratings that online users have applied to retailers. These are usually stars (usually up to 5 stars, and the more stars the better). Many of the shopping portals in the previous section also include user ratings for each store. For example, Google Product Search (www.google.com/products/) also doubles as a retailer ratings service. When you run a product search, the name of the seller appears below the price—and below that are a rating (1 to 5 stars) and the number of user ratings that have produced the result. As you can see in Figure 13.4, you can also sort the results by seller rating.

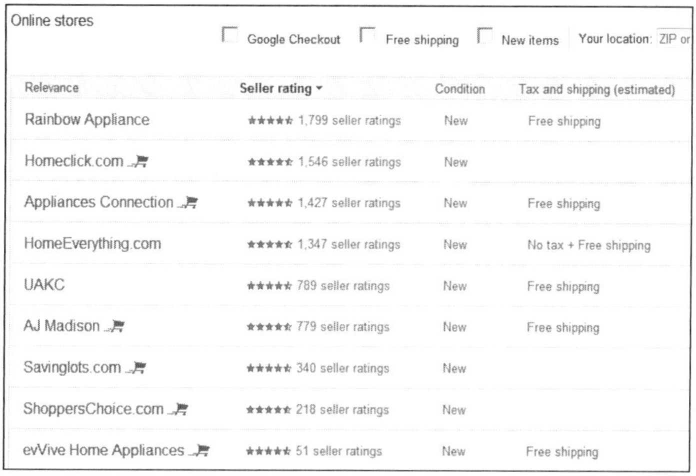

Online stores			
☐ Google Checkout ☐ Free shipping ☐ New items Your location: ZIP or			
Relevance	Seller rating ▼	Condition	Tax and shipping (estimated)
Rainbow Appliance	★★★★★ 1,799 seller ratings	New	Free shipping
Homeclick.com	★★★★★ 1,546 seller ratings	New	
Appliances Connection	★★★★★ 1,427 seller ratings	New	Free shipping
HomeEverything.com	★★★★★ 1,347 seller ratings	New	No tax + Free shipping
UAKC	★★★★★ 789 seller ratings	New	Free shipping
AJ Madison	★★★★★ 779 seller ratings	New	Free shipping
Savinglots.com	★★★★★ 340 seller ratings	New	
ShoppersChoice.com	★★★★★ 218 seller ratings	New	
evVive Home Appliances	★★★★★ 51 seller ratings	New	Free shipping

Figure 13.4: You can sort the Google Product Search results by seller rating.

A site that's dedicated to rating resellers is the appropriately named ResellerRatings.com (www.resellerratings.com). This site uses a 1-to-10 scale, where the higher the rating, the better the store. You can use the site as a shopping portal, or you can look up an individual store to see its rating. (Usually, you get 2 ratings for each store: a lifetime rating and a 6-month rating; if the latter is much lower than the former, that's a sign something has gone seriously wrong at the store over the last few months and you may want to shop elsewhere.) There are also interesting lists of the "Best Stores" (see Figure 13.5) and "Worst Stores."

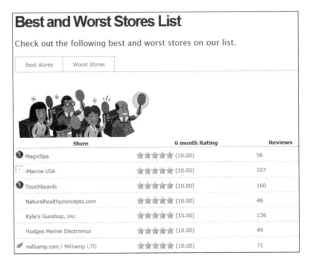

Figure 13.5: ResellerRatings.com is a massive database of online retailer ratings and reviews.

Buying Things Online

Buying products online isn't the scary proposition it was a few years ago. There are many reliable, reputable, and secure merchants to choose from now, so buying online is no longer a big deal. Even still, it's different from buying at a retail store or via mail order. To ensure the best online transaction possible, see the tips in Chapter 17 on preventing fraud while shopping online, and bear in mind the following pointers:

- The three most important things to remember when buying online are compare, compare, compare. It's not at all unusual to find one store selling the same item for 10 percent or even 20 percent less than other stores, so use the shopping portals I mentioned earlier to get the best price.

- Keep an eye out for special deals. Many online retailers offer promotions on a particular day of the week or when they need to clear out inventory. Troll the sites of your favorite online retailers to watch out for these specials.

- Buy just off the bleeding edge. If you're buying a computer, computer accessories, consumer electronics, or just about any kind of digital doodad, it's a truism that the latest-and-greatest parts cost the most. A company's brand-new digital camera may run $800 to $1,000, but last year's model, which is a perfectly good camera, may sell for half that.

- When the checkout process is complete, leave the final window open on your desktop so you have access to the order number, the final total, tracking information, and other details. After you get an email confirming the transaction and you've checked the email for accuracy, you can close the web window.

Good to Know!

In the unlikely event that the retailer doesn't provide a confirmation email message, either print the screen or capture it to an image. For the latter, press the **Print Screen** key (it may be labeled **Prt Scr** or something equally obscure), then paste the image into the Paint program.

Booking a Trip

If you have the "urge for going" (as the song says), there are plenty of online resources that can help make it happen.

Once you have a destination in mind, you'll want to get some advice on the best time to go, how to get there, where to stay, how to get around, places to visit, and so on. The web can help here because it offers tons of trip-planning resources. Here's a sampling (Figure 13.6 shows the Expedia site):

- **Expedia** www.expedia.com
- **Flight Center** www.flightcenter.com

- **Orbitz**   www.orbitz.com
- **TripAdvisor**   www.tripadvisor.com
- **Travelocity**   www.travelocity.com

By the Way

When you try to access these sites, you may get bumped to a similar site with a slightly different address. That's because most of these sites offer country-specific versions of their websites. So, for example, if you try to access expedia.com from Canada, you end up at expedia.ca, the site version optimized for Canadian users.

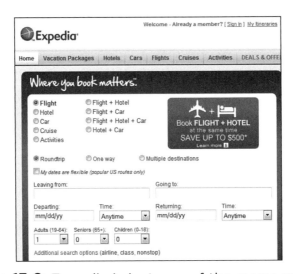

Figure 13.6: Expedia is just one of the many excellent trip-planning sites on the web.

Most of these trip-planning sites (Expedia, Flight Center, Orbitz, and Travelocity) are also happy to book your flight for you. This is often the best way to get a good deal, because these services have access to insider deals and can negotiate lower prices. However, airlines often offer special deals to customers who book directly with them (and they're often a lot quicker to help you if something goes awry with your flights), so it pays to check with the airlines to make sure you're getting the best deal. All the major airlines are online (for example, Figure 13.7 shows the Delta Airlines site: www.delta.com), so a quick Bing or Google search will locate any carrier you want to check out.

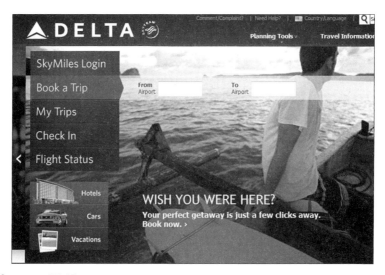

Figure 13.7: Delta is just one of hundreds of airlines that have colonized the web.

Also, here are three sites that can help you find the right seat on the right flight for the right price:

- **Airfare Watchdog (www.airfarewatchdog.com)** This site tells you about airline sales and flight deals and even lets you sign up for email alerts when there are low fares departing from your location.

- **Priceline (www.priceline.com)** This site is the famous and popular discount airfare purveyor.

- **SeatGuru (www.seatguru.com)**   This website offers maps of the seating on each flight and can advise you on the best seats to choose. (In fact, *Time* magazine named SeatGuru one of its 50 Best Websites for 2010.)

When you're ready to book your hotel room, first check to see whether your travel agent or trip-planning service offers combined flight and hotel deals (which can save you some money). However, you can also sometimes eke out a good deal by dealing with the hotel directly. All the larger chains and the vast majority of smaller and boutique hotels have websites these days, so take a look around for special deals and upcoming events.

Finally, if cruising is your style, the web offers lots of useful resources for researching, locating, and booking your trip. All the major cruise lines have websites, although there are significant differences in terms of interaction with customers, promotions, and other goodies.

Using Online Coupons

You probably know that using coupons in the real world can save you enough pennies here and there to add up to some serious dollars. Fortunately, you can also export that same satisfying frugality to the web world by taking advantage of online coupons. There are three main types to consider: coupon codes, printable coupons, and group coupons.

Probably the most common type of online coupon is the *coupon code* (sometimes called a *promotional code*). This is usually a numeric code or some combination of letters and numbers that you specify when you're completing a purchase online, and it tells the merchant to give you a special deal (such as 10 percent off your purchase).

How do you get a coupon code? It may come in a marketing email message if you've asked the company to send you such things. However, there are also sites that list hundreds or thousands of coupon codes for a wide variety of online retailers. Here are a few to get you started (Figure 13.8 shows the RetailMeNot site):

- **Coupon Cabin**   www.couponcabin.com
- **Coupon Mom**   www.couponmom.com
- **Coupon Shack**   www.couponshack.com
- **Current Codes**   www.currentcodes.com
- **Grocery Coupon Network**   www.grocerycouponnetwork.com
- **Promotional Codes**   www.promotionalcodes.com
- **RetailMeNot**   www.retailmenot.com

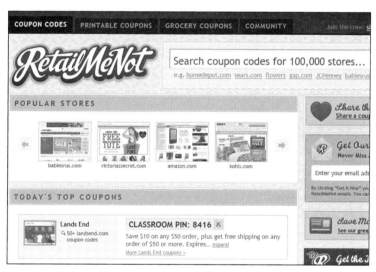

Figure 13.8: RetailMeNot is the most popular of the many coupon-code sites on the web.

The second most common type of online coupon is the *printable coupon*, which is pretty much what you'd expect: an image of a coupon that you print out and then take to the store, just like a regular paper coupon. Most of the coupon sites I listed earlier also come with printable coupon sections. Another good source is the website of the retailer. For example, almost all major grocery chains offer printable coupons at least some of the time.

The third type of online coupon is the *group coupon*, which offers a discount or similar deal, but only if a specified minimum number of people commit to the purchase. For example, consider the group coupon deal shown in Figure 13.9. This is for a facial, and the price is $37, which is a 51 percent discount from the regular price of $75. So far, 13 people have committed to purchasing the facial, but the retailer has specified that a minimum number of 15 people must be in on the purchase—so two more are needed. You also see that the deal expires in about 1 day and 7 hours. What happens if the time period ends and the minimum number of people haven't signed up? The deal expires, and no money changes hands.

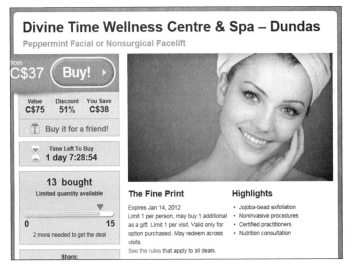

Figure 13.9: With a group coupon, a deal isn't a deal until a minimum number of people commit to it.

Group coupons are a hot item these days, and sites are popping up all over the place—although most cover only a small number of cities. As I write this, there are two major players in the group coupon scene (the deal shown in Figure 13.9 is from the Groupon site):

- **Groupon**   www.groupon.com
- **LivingSocial**   www.livingsocial.com

The Least You Need to Know

- Online shopping saves time and gas, offers a large selection, and makes comparison shopping a breeze, but it also means you can't touch or try on products, shipping fees can be exorbitant, and it takes a day or three to get your stuff.
- There are many sites online that enable you to research products, prices, and retailers, so be sure to take advantage of these useful resources.
- Look for deals that are good but not *too* good. Also, remember to enter your ZIP or postal code so you know what the shipping fees will be.
- To save even more money online, look for coupon codes, printable coupons, and group coupons.

Chapter 14

Connecting with Family and Friends

In This Chapter

- Getting a grip on the social-networking thing
- Determining which social network is best for you
- Figuring out Facebook
- Making "friends" and sharing information

Social networking is one of the internet's most popular pastimes, with some sites boasting millions of members. When you join a social network, you can connect with other people and then use those connections to send messages, share the latest news and updates, exchange photos and website links, and much more.

In this chapter, you find out what social networking is all about and learn some details about Facebook, the most popular social-networking site.

Understanding Social Networking

Social networking has been around for only a few years, but it's already the most popular and most-talked-about internet pastime. Before you take the social-networking plunge, you should spend a few minutes to understand what this phenomenon is all about. What, exactly, is the point of social networking? What's all this about "friends"? What types of information and data can you share with those friends? What kinds of privacy and security issues come up when you share your data online?

> **Definition**
>
> **Social networking** is an internet service that enables you to share information with family, friends, and people who have similar hobbies and interests.

For starters, there are a couple main reasons why people use social-networking sites. First, these sites are an easy and convenient way to keep track of what's going on in the lives of friends, family, and acquaintances—particularly people who you don't see regularly. Second, social-networking sites are a great way to expand your circle of friends and contacts, because you can usually see and connect with the friends of your existing friends—and you can also see or find other people who share your interests.

All social-networking sites give everyone limited access to the site's features and members. However, if you want to access all the site's features—and in particular, if you want to connect with the site's members—then you must sign up for an account. All social-networking sites offer free membership (they earn their money by displaying advertisements), and the sign-up process usually requests a limited amount of personal data, including your name, a display name that others see, your email address, and your location.

All social networks revolve around the concept of friends (sometimes called followers or connections). A friend is another member of the same social network that you have established a relationship with. In most cases, you establish this relationship by sending the person a friend request. If the other person accepts the request, he or she is added to your list of friends. This enables you to send messages to that person, view that person's profile, and see his or her status updates.

When you become a member of a social-networking site, one of the first things you usually do is fill in your personal profile. The information in this profile varies from site to site, but the data usually includes your interests and hobbies, your current and past jobs, your education, your birthday, your relationship status, and a photo.

Making friends is the "networking" part of social networking, and the "social" part involves sharing information and data with your friends. What information and how you share it depends on the site, but in most cases you can share things such as updates on your current status or activities, photos, groups on the site that you have joined, blog posts, and links to interesting sites on the World Wide Web.

If you are concerned about making so much personal information available online, remember that in most cases you can add to your profile only the information that you are comfortable sharing with others. Also, all social networks come with privacy features that enable you to control who gets to see your stuff.

Finding the Right Social Network

The bad news about social networks is that there are just so darned many of them. There are, distressingly, *hundreds*—perhaps even *thousands*—of them infesting the internet. Fortunately, the vast majority of these social networks are either so-called "niche" networks—meaning they're focused on a specific topic, such as parenting, music, or knitting—or they're popular only in certain countries. For example, Google's original social network is called Orkut, and for some reason it's only popular now in Brazil.

> **By the Way**
>
> Yes, I said *knitting*. Actually, the site I'm thinking of is called Ravelry (www.ravelry.com), and by all accounts it's a fantastic social network if you're into knitting, crocheting, or weaving. It's amazingly popular, too, with nearly 1.5 million members.

So the *good* news is that you can ignore almost all the social networks out there and concentrate on only the most useful and popular ones—which, by happy coincidence, are probably also the ones that your family members and friends are using. Here they are:

- **Facebook (www.facebook.com)**   This is, by far, the most popular social network, with more than 750 million members. It's extremely popular with seniors (in fact, the 65-plus group is the fastest-growing demographic on Facebook), and chances are that many of your family members have Facebook accounts (and quite a few of your friends will have beaten you there, as well). With Facebook, you friend (yes, it's also a verb) other people and then exchange news, links, photos, and videos; play games; and explore the wealth of resources that Facebook's members have created.

- **Twitter (www.twitter.com)**   This is the next most popular social network, with more than 200 million members. Twitter is all about sharing short text messages—called *tweets*—that, famously, can be no more than 140 characters. With Twitter, you "follow" other people, which enables you to see their tweets—and other people follow you to see your tweets.

- **Google+ (http://plus.google.com/)**   This is the new kid on the social-networking block. Google+ is similar to Facebook, but it gives you more control over who sees the information you share. For example, you can organize people into separate groups called "circles," and you can then share things like status updates and photos only with people in a particular circle.

- **LinkedIn (www.linkedin.com)**   This is a very popular social network, with more than 100 million members. LinkedIn's focus is business relationships, and through your connections you can look for professionals to work with (and other professionals can find you). This is only a good social network for you if you're working.

- **MySpace (www.myspace.com)** This was the top social network a couple years ago, but it has fallen out of favor since then. Still, it does boast about 30 million members, so you may have kids (or, more likely, grandkids) on the site. MySpace members tend to be quite young, so steer clear unless you know a few people on the site.

So which social network is right for you? If you only want to join one network, then Facebook is a no-brainer because it's so popular and enables you to do and share so many things. If you feel that Facebook is too public, though, Twitter may be more to your liking because you don't have to use your real name—and you can share just the information that you're comfortable sharing. Note, too, that you can use both if you have the time; lots of people do so because Facebook and Twitter are quite different.

> **By the Way**
>
> Yes, there are social networks designed for seniors, and you're free to give one or more of them a whirl to see whether any are right for you. The most popular are AARP Online Community (www.aarp.org/online_community/), Eons (www.eons.com), and My Boomer Place (www.myboomerplace.com).

Setting Up and Using a Facebook Account

Social networks are all about making connections, and it's certainly true that any social network will enable you to make friends with or follow people you don't know who share your interests, tastes, or sense of humor. However, when you're just starting with social networking, it's natural to begin by making connections with people you *do* know—particularly family, friends, old work colleagues, or even school chums from back in the day.

Finding people you know is often difficult on smaller social networks, but it's unlikely to be a problem on Facebook. With three quarters of a *billion* people now using Facebook, you're pretty much guaranteed to be surrounded by a herd of familiar faces. This section shows you how to get started with Facebook, how to configure your profile, how to make friends, and then how to share news, photos, and links.

Creating a Facebook Account

To use Facebook, you need to create an account (there's no charge). Let's begin by going through the necessary steps:

1. Surf to www.facebook.com.

2. In the Sign Up section, fill in your name, your email address (twice), a password for your account, your gender, and your birth date, as shown in Figure 14.1.

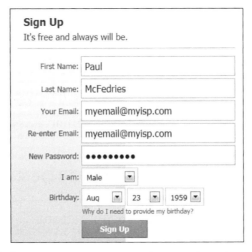

Figure 14.1: To get started with Facebook, go to www.facebook.com and fill in the Sign Up section.

3. Click **Sign Up**. Facebook displays the Security Check page, which it needs to prevent scammers and other undesirables from using automated systems to create Facebook accounts.

4. Type the words you see in the box, then click **Sign Up**. Facebook prompts you to look for friends who are already using the service.

What Can Go Wrong?

If you can't read the words, click the **Try different words** link until you get a set of words that you can decipher. If your eyesight just isn't up to the task, click the **audio captcha** link instead to hear the words spoken.

5. I'll show you how to find your existing friends in the next section, so click **Skip this step** to keep things moving. Facebook prompts you to fill in some profile information.

6. Again, we'll get into all that after these steps are done, so click **Skip** to keep going. Facebook now prompts you to set your profile picture.

7. We'll get there eventually, so click **Skip** yet again. Facebook takes you to your account but lets you know that it has sent a confirmation message to your email account.

8. Open your email program, click the Facebook message (it's the one with the Subject line, "Just one more step to get started on Facebook"), and then click the link that appears in the message (or click the **Complete Sign-up** button).

With all that out of the way, your Facebook account is ready to roll, and you see a page similar to the one shown in Figure 14.2.

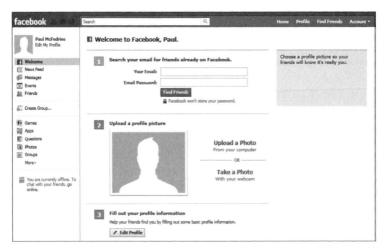

Figure 14.2: Once you click the link in the confirmation email, your Facebook account is ready for action.

Configuring Your Facebook Profile

Before you go any further with Facebook, you should take a step back and fill in some details in your profile. As I mentioned earlier, you don't have to share *everything* about yourself, but Facebook is more interesting and more fun if you at least share a little. Let's give it a whirl:

1. Click the **Edit My Profile** link in the upper-left corner of the Welcome to Facebook page. This launches the Edit Profile page, shown in Figure 14.3.

2. The Basic Information section comes up first, so use this section to fill in some general data about yourself, then click **Save Changes**.

3. If you want to show off a picture of your smiling (or not) mug, click **Profile Picture**, and then click either **Browse** to choose a picture file from your computer or click **Take a Picture** if your computer has a camera attached.

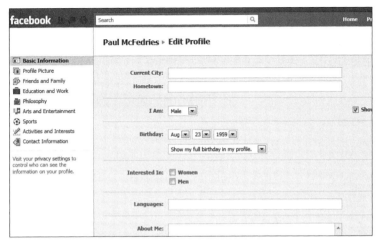

Figure 14.3: Use the Edit Profile page to specify the information you want to share with people on Facebook.

4. Work your way through the rest of the sections—Friends and Family, Education and Work, Activities and Interests, and so on—and fill in as much information as you feel comfortable sharing. Remember to click **Save Changes** in each section before moving on to the next section.

5. When you're done, click **Home** near the top of the page to return to your Facebook homepage.

Making Friends

You can certainly do lots of things on Facebook without connecting with other people. For example, you can use the Search box at the top of the page to look for interesting Facebook pages, and you can use the Games and Apps links on the left side of the page to play games and work with Facebook applications.

However, to get the most from Facebook, you really need to make some connections with people. On Facebook, this is called *friending* people, and the resulting connections are called *friends*. (Note that Facebook uses the word "friend" not only for actual friends but also for family members, old colleagues, acquaintances, and even complete strangers, if it comes to that.)

Facebook offers three main ways to locate people you want to friend: individually, by affiliation (such as company name or school name), or by contacts list.

Here's how to search for a particular person on Facebook:

1. Click inside the **Search** text box at the top of the screen.

2. Type the person's name or email address. Facebook displays a list of matching resources, as shown in Figure 14.4.

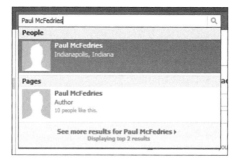

Figure 14.4: Use the Search box to look for a person you want to friend.

3. If you see the person you want, click that list item, and then skip to step 6. If you don't see the person you want or if you're not sure, click the **See more results** link at the bottom of the list.

4. Click **People** on the left side of the window.

5. If you see someone who you think is your friend, click that person in the list to bring up that person's Facebook profile page. If it's not the right person, click the browser's **Back** button and try again.

6. Click **Add Friend**. Facebook asks you to confirm, as shown in Figure 14.5.

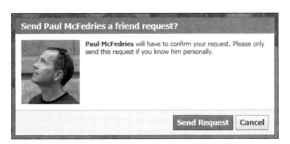

Figure 14.5: Click **Add Friend**, then click **Send Request** to send your friend invitation.

7. Click **Send Request**. Facebook lets the other person know about your friend request, and that person will then either accept or reject the request (hopefully the former!).

To look for current or former work colleagues or old college or high school classmates, follow these steps:

1. Click **Home** near the top of the page.

2. Click **Friends** on the left side of the page.

3. Near the bottom of the page, click **Other Tools** and then click **Find Friends, Classmates, and Coworkers**.

4. To look for people by location, fill in either the **Hometown** or **Current City** field.

5. To look for people by affiliation, fill in the **High School**, **College or University**, **Employer**, or **Graduate School** field.

6. In the list that appears, click a person to check out his or her Facebook profile page. If it's not the right person, click the browser's **Back** button and try again.

7. Click **Add Friend**. Facebook asks you to confirm.

8. Click **Send Request**.

Finally, Facebook is on friendly (so to speak) terms with a number of web-based email services, including Hotmail and Yahoo!. If you use one of these services, you can provide Facebook with your email address. Facebook prompts you to log in to your account, and then it grabs your contact list from the service and lets you know whether any of your contacts are already on Facebook.

Good to Know!

Give my email password to Facebook? Am I crazy? The state of my mental health is occasionally up for debate, but in this case I'm being quite sane. Facebook actually doesn't see your password because the login occurs through your email service.

Follow these steps to look for potential Facebook friends through your email service's contacts list:

1. Click **Home** near the top of the page.

2. Click **Friends** on the left side of the page.

3. Click the email service you use.

4. Type your email address, then click **Find Friends**. Facebook connects with your email service, and that service asks you to log in to your account.

5. Type your password, and then click **Sign In** (or **Log In**, or whatever).

6. With some services, you have to agree to allow Facebook to access your account, so click **Agree** (or whatever) to make it so. Facebook grabs your contacts and displays a list of those who are on Facebook, as shown in Figure 14.6.

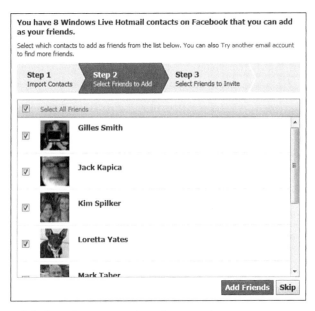

Figure 14.6: After Facebook convinces your email service to send your contacts list, it then tells you who is already on Facebook.

7. Deactivate the check box beside any person you don't want to friend.

8. Click **Add Friends**. Facebook sends the friend requests, then presents you with a list of your contacts who aren't on Facebook so you can invite them to join.

9. These invitations are a tad presumptuous and a little annoying, so you'd do well to steer clear here. Click **Skip** to save your friendships.

Handling a Friend Request

Of course, while you're busy looking for people on Facebook, people on Facebook may be busy looking for *you!* If they find you, then you can expect a friend request or two to come your way.

How do you know? The next time you log in to your Facebook account, take a look in the upper-left corner of the page, beside the Facebook logo. If you see a small red icon with a white number inside beside the Friends icon (the one with the two heads), as shown in Figure 14.7, it means you have a friend request. (The number inside the icon tells you how many requests are waiting.)

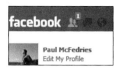

Figure 14.7: When a friend request comes in, you see a red icon with a number beside the Friends icon.

Click the **Friends** icon to see who made the request, as shown in Figure 14.8, then click **Confirm** if you want to be friends with this person (or **Not Now** if you don't).

> **By the Way**
>
> There are two things to remember about clicking Not Now for a friend request. First, the other person never knows that you've clicked Not Now, so you won't hurt anyone's feelings; second, Facebook merely hides the friend request, it doesn't reject it outright. If you change your mind, click **Home**, click **Friends**, and then click **See X Hidden Requests** (where *X* is the number of people you've put off with the Not Now button).

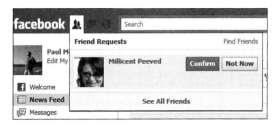

Figure 14.8: Click the **Friends** icon to see who made the friend request, and then click either **Confirm** or **Not Now**.

Update Your Status on Facebook

Once you're friends with at least one person, click **News Feed** on the left side to see a list of the most recent Facebook activities of your friends. These activities include friending other people, commenting on things their friends are doing, sharing photos and links, and much more. The News Feed also includes your friends' latest status updates. A status update is a simple text message that aims to reflect whatever is on your mind. It could be something you've just done (or are doing); a favorite quotation; something clever, wise, or pithy you just thought of; a question; or a comment about something.

Follow these steps to update your Facebook status:

1. Click **Home** at the top of the page. Facebook displays your News Feed.
2. Click **Status**. (Actually, this is almost always selected by default, so you can probably skip this step.)
3. Click inside the **What's on your mind?** text box.
4. Type your status update.
5. Click the **Privacy** icon (see Figure 14.9), and then click who can see your updates. The default is Everyone, but you may want to choose Friends Only to limit who can see your update.

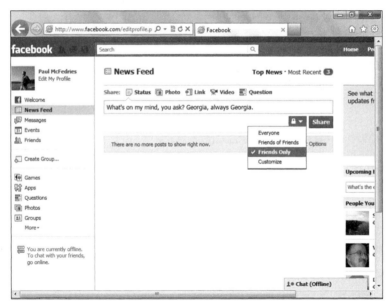

Figure 14.9: Click **Status**, type your update, and then use the Privacy icon to set who can see it.

6. Click **Share**. Facebook updates your status, and the new status appears in the News Feed of each of your friends.

Share Photos on Facebook

One of the most popular pastimes on Facebook is sharing photos with your friends. It's certainly a great deal easier than printing out and sending a photo, and it's even easier than emailing a photo because Facebook lets you share the photo with a large number of people instantly.

Follow these steps to share a photo with your Facebook friends:

1. Click **Home** at the top of the page. Facebook displays your News Feed.
2. Click **Photo**.
3. Click **Upload a Photo**.
4. Click **Browse**.
5. Select the photo you want to share, then click **Open**.
6. Click inside the **Say something about this photo** text box.
7. Type a description, comment, or something else about the photo.
8. Click the **Privacy** icon to choose who can see your photo.
9. Click **Share**. Facebook shares the photo, which then appears in the News Feed of each of your friends.

Share Links on Facebook

If you come across an interesting, funny, or useful website, why not tell your Facebook friends about it? Follow these steps to share a link on Facebook:

1. Use Internet Explorer to navigate to the site you want to share.
2. Right-click the site address in the Address bar, then click **Copy**.
3. In Facebook, click **Home** at the top of the page. Facebook displays your News Feed.

4. Click **Link**.

5. Click inside the **http://** text box.

6. Press **Ctrl+V** to paste the address into the text box.

7. Click **Attach**. If Facebook mumbles something about everyone being able to see the link, click **Continue**.

8. Click inside the **Say something about this link** text box.

9. Type a description, comment, or something else about the link.

10. Click the **Privacy** icon, then click who can see your link.

11. Click **Share**. Facebook shares the link, which then appears in the News Feed of each of your friends.

The Least You Need to Know

- A social network is an internet service that enables you to share updates, photos, and other information with family members, friends, and people who have similar hobbies and interests.
- Social-networking sites are an easy and convenient way to keep track of what's going on in the lives of friends and family—especially folks you don't see very often.
- In social networking, a "friend" is another member of the same social network that you have established a relationship with.
- Facebook and Twitter are the most popular social networks. If you're primarily interested in connecting with family and friends, then Facebook is your best choice.
- To create a Facebook account, go to www.facebook.com and fill in your details.
- To share information with your Facebook friends, click **Home**, then click **Status**, **Photo**, or **Link**.

Staying Safe Online

Part 4

The internet is a more cosmopolitan place now than in its relatively lawless beginnings. However, although the internet is no longer the digital equivalent of the Wild West, we've progressed only to about the level of, say, New York City in the 1970s. That is to say, the internet is a fun and fascinating place with an impressive number of things to see and do—but there are parts of town that it's best to avoid.

Fortunately, the situation is not so grim that you can't easily protect yourself. As you'll see in Part 4, avoiding viruses, spam, scams, and other internet unpleasantness is a relatively simple combination of common sense and the prudent tweaking of a few settings.

Playing It Safe on the Web

Chapter **15**

In This Chapter

- Guarding against viruses
- Protecting yourself from spyware
- Using credit cards securely
- Keeping your surfing sessions private
- Blocking those annoying pop-up windows

The web is one of the Seven Wonders of the Modern World. (The others, in case you're wondering, are the smartphone, the electric car, the CN Tower, the Aeron office chair, the Global Positioning System, and Donald Trump's hair.) The web earns that honor by being the world's ultimate trove of knowledge, information, facts, entertainment, and sheer fun. However, it would be a mistake to think of the web as a kind of digital Shangri-La where bad things never happen to good people. The web is a reflection of life, and as such it can also reflect the bad side. So, unfortunately, the web is home to people who'd like to take over your computer, steal your credit card data, grab your online banking password, and generally just cause whatever mischief and mayhem they think they can get away with.

Fortunately, these digital ne'er-do-wells are relatively rare, so it's not like you're going to be constantly accosted as you travel around the internet.

But e-hooligans do exist, so the prudent web surfer understands the potential threats and takes steps to prevent bad things from happening. This chapter tells you everything you need to know to stay safe when you're on the web.

Avoiding Viruses

A *virus* is a software program that installs on your computer surreptitiously. Some viruses are relatively benign and only display annoying messages—but most viruses are designed for nefarious purposes, such as stealing or deleting data, crashing your computer, or hijacking your PC to attack other computers.

> **Definition**
>
> A **virus** is a software program that installs itself on your computer without you knowing it, then proceeds to steal or destroy data or crash or hijack your computer.

To prevent viruses from infecting your computer, you need to install an *antivirus program*. This is a special software program that maintains a list of known viruses as well as the means to block those viruses. This virus list is crucial, and it's constantly being updated (because unfortunately, new viruses are constantly being created)—so be sure to keep your antivirus program's virus list up-to-date. (The good news? Most antivirus programs do this automatically.) Here are some security suites to check out:

- Avast! Antivirus (www.avast.com)
- AVG Internet Security (http://free.grisoft.com/)
- McAfee Internet Security Suite (www.mcafee.com)
- Norton Internet Security (http://us.norton.com/)

Note that AVG Internet Security is free, but the others require annual payments to keep their virus definitions up to date.

Even after you've installed your antivirus program, you still need to keep your wits about you while wandering the web to avoid the hassle of dealing with a virus. Specifically, you need to watch out for the following:

- **Links to potentially dangerous files.** By "potentially dangerous," I mean what computer nerds call "executable" files, which just means files that launch a program or script. That's potentially dangerous because such a file could be launching a program that installs a virus on your system. Before clicking a link, take a look at the bottom of the web browser window to see the link address. Don't click the link if the file name ends with any of the following codes: .bat, .cmd, .com, .doc, .exe, .js, .ppt, .reg, .vb, .vbs, .wsh, or .xls.

- **Files from sites you don't know or don't trust.** Files that come from reputable websites are almost certainly virus-free. However, if you download a file from a site you don't know or trust, you should use your antivirus software to scan the file for infection before opening it.

- **Ads that make bold or hyperbolic claims.** If you see a website ad that tells you that you have messages waiting or that you've won a prize, don't believe it. And particularly, don't click anything inside the ad or you may cause a virus to be installed. For some real chutzpah, nothing beats an ad that tells you your system is infected (see Figure 15.1), instructs you to click something to fix the problem, and then proceeds to infect your system!

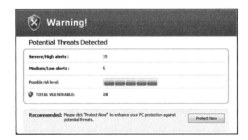

Figure 15.1: If you see a warning that your system is infected, run the other way!

- **Pop-up windows that won't go away.** The ads that I talked about in the previous item also appear in pop-up windows, which are separate web browser windows that appear suddenly on your screen when you access a site. Again, avoid clicking anything inside a pop-up window, because that could trigger the virus installation.

When I say, "Avoid clicking anything within a pop-up window," I mean *anything*. Even something as seemingly innocuous as a red "X" button that looks just like a Close button may not be safe. So how do you close a pop-up window? Here are three methods to try:

- Press **Ctrl+W**.
- Click the Internet Explorer icon in the taskbar to display thumbnail versions of the open windows, right-click the thumbnail of the pop-up window, and then click **Close**.
- If none of these methods work, right-click the taskbar, click **Start Task Manager**, click the pop-up window in the Applications tab's list of running programs, and then click **End Task**.

Keeping Spyware at Bay

If you access the internet using a broadband cable modem or digital subscriber line (DSL) service, chances are you have an "always-on" connection—which means there's a much greater chance that a malicious hacker could find your computer and have his or her way with it. You may think that with hundreds of millions of people connected to the internet at any given moment, there would be little chance of a nefarious user finding you in the herd. Unfortunately, one of the most common weapons in the arsenal of your typical cracker (a malicious hacker) is a program that runs through millions of addresses automatically, looking for "live" connections. The problem is compounded by the fact that many cable systems and some DSL systems use addresses in a narrow range, thus making it easier to find always-on connections.

However, having a hacker locate your system isn't a big deal as long as he or she can't get into your system. There are two ways to prevent this: one is to turn on Windows Firewall, which blocks unauthorized access to your computer and is (thankfully) activated by default in Windows 7; the other is to take steps to avoid accidentally letting a hacker into your system.

Good to Know!

It pays to take a second and check that Windows Firewall is actually on the job. Select **Start**, **Control Panel**, **System and Security**, **Check firewall status**. In the Windows Firewall window, make sure the Windows Firewall state shows On. If it doesn't, click **Turn Windows Firewall on or off** and then select **Turn on Windows Firewall**.

In recent years, a new threat to our PCs has emerged. It's called *spyware*, and it's a nasty bit of digital business that threatens to deprive a significant portion of the online world of their sanity. Spyware refers to a program that surreptitiously monitors your computer activities—particularly the typing of passwords, personal identification numbers (PINs), and credit card numbers—or harvests sensitive data on your computer, then sends that information to an individual or a company via your internet connection.

You may think that having Windows Firewall between you and the bad guys would make spyware a problem of the past. Unfortunately, that's not true. These programs piggyback on other legitimate programs that you actually *want* to download, such as file-sharing programs, download managers, and screen savers. To make matters even worse, most spyware embeds itself deep into a system—and removing it is a delicate and time-consuming operation beyond the abilities of even most experienced users. Some programs actually come with an "uninstall" option, but it's nothing but a ruse, of course. The program appears to remove itself from the system, but what it actually does is reinstall a fresh version of itself when the computer is idle.

All this means that you need to buttress Windows Firewall with an antispyware program that can watch out for these unwanted programs and prevent them from getting their hooks into your system. Happily, Windows 7 comes with just such a program, and it has an appropriate (and hopefully accurate!) name: Windows Defender.

Out of the box, Windows 7 sets up Windows Defender to protect your system from spyware nastiness in two ways:

- Windows Defender scans your system for spyware infestations every day at 2 A.M.
- Windows Defender runs in the background full-time to watch out for spyware-like activity. If it detects a spyware fiend trying to sneak in the back door, Windows Defender terminates the brute with extreme prejudice.

Good to Know!

Windows Defender can only scan your computer if it's running, which is a problem if you turn off your computer at night. To work around this, you can change the time when Windows Defender runs the scan. Click **Start**, type **defend**, and then click **Windows Defender** in the search results. Click **Tools**, click **Options**, and then use the Approximate time list to choose a time when your computer is on.

As with Windows Firewall, what you need to do is check to make sure that both of these protection features are turned on. Here's how:

1. Click **Start**, type **defend** in the Start menu's Search box, and then click **Windows Defender** in the search results.

2. Select **Tools** to display the Tools and Settings window.

3. Select **Options** to open the Options window.

By the Way

Feel free to run a scan on your computer right now if you like. Launch Windows Defender and then click **Scan** to do a quick scan. If you want a more thorough check, pull down the **Scan** list and select **Full Scan**.

4. Select **Automatic scanning** and then activate the **Automatically scan my computer** check box. While you're here, you can also monkey with the scan schedule (**Frequency**, **Approximate time**, and **Type**).

5. Select **Real-time protection**, then activate the **Use real-time protection** check box.

6. Click **Save**.

Heeding Windows's Warnings

You may have noticed while traipsing around the Windows 7 landscape that from time to time, the system asks for permission to perform some task. Why the persnicketiness? It's all about security.

As the main user of your computer, you have lots of power over the system. That's not a bad thing on its own, but the social misfits who create viruses and other malicious programs found ways to take advantage of the situation. Specifically, if you were logged on to Windows and a virus leeched into your system, that virus would have complete access to the system—and that almost always spelled disaster.

So the famously big brains at Microsoft figured out a way to thwart viruses and their ilk. It's called *user account control* (UAC), and in a nutshell it means that users no longer have complete run of the system. Sure, they can still do all the things they used to, but now they have to provide credentials to Windows to, in a sense, prove that they're not a virus. How you provide those credentials depends on the type of user account you're logged on with:

- If you're an administrator (that is, the main user), you see the User Account Control dialog box shown in Figure 15.2. In this case, all you have to do is click **Yes** to proceed with whatever you wanted to do.

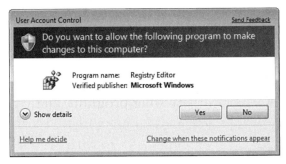

Figure 15.2: If you're an administrator, Windows 7 displays this dialog box when it needs your permission to perform some action.

- If you're a standard user, you see the User Account Control dialog box shown in Figure 15.3 instead. Windows shows the name of the original computer administrator (you may see other administrator accounts, if your computer has them) and prompts you for that user's password. After you type the administrator's password, click **Yes** to continue on your way.

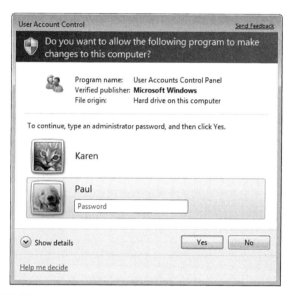

Figure 15.3: If you're a standard user, Windows displays this dialog box when it needs your permission to perform some action.

Secure Surfing: Some General Tips

Land on the wrong website, and a malicious script may do something nasty to your PC; install the wrong program, and you may end up with spyware or a virus installed right along with it; type your email address in the wrong place, and you may end up with even more spam than you have already.

How's a body to bypass these threats and still enjoy the online world? Fortunately, it's not that hard. Besides installing an antivirus program and ensuring that Windows Defender is on the job, you can also do a few more general things:

- **Keep your PC** *patched*. Your worst enemy when it comes to online safety is actually your operating system! The sheer number of Windows vulnerabilities is staggering, and the only chance you have to prevent some hacker from taking advantage of just one of those holes is to apply any and all security-related updates that Microsoft releases.

> **Definition**
>
> To **patch** your PC means to install any and all Windows updates that Microsoft makes available.

- **Load up your machine with anti-malware**. Windows Defender is a good program, but no antispyware program can stop all spyware. To ensure that all your holes are filled, adding a second antispyware program wouldn't hurt. The security suites I mentioned come with antispyware components, but you can also check out Ad-Aware (www.lavasoft.com), Spyware Doctor (www.pctools.com), and Spybot Search & Destroy (www.safer-networking.org).

- **Pay attention, and use common sense**. Lots of people run into trouble online, not because cyberspace is an inherently dangerous place but because the vast majority of those people simply weren't paying attention to what they were doing. If an offer sounds too good to be true, it almost certainly is. If a file attachment shows up unexpectedly, it probably contains something unexpected (and unwelcome). If Windows's User Account Control dialog box shows up without you doing anything, it means that something *else* is doing something, and it's correct to assume that it's up to no good.

Windows can't do much to ensure that your store of common sense is topped up, but it can help you with your PC's update and anti-malware status. The Windows Action Center offers a quick peek at your security settings and shows you right away if anything's amiss. To launch the Windows Action Center, select **Start**, **Control Panel**, and then under the **System and Security** heading, click **Review your computer's status and resolve issues**.

In Windows Vista, select **Start**, **Control Panel**, and then under the **Security** heading, click **Check this computer's security status**. In Windows XP, select **Start**, **Control Panel**, **Security Center**.

Figure 15.4 shows the Action Center window with a couple problems. In this case, this PC has an out-of-date version of Windows Defender and no antivirus program installed.

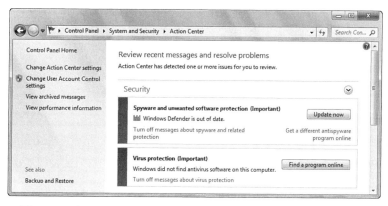

Figure 15.4: Drop in on the Action Center to see whether Windows has any security concerns about your computer.

Even More Ways to Protect Yourself on the Web

Okay, so now you're watching out for viruses and spyware, you're looking twice (perhaps even three times) at website ads and pop-up windows, and you've promised to pay attention whenever the User Account Control dialog box drops by for a chat. That should be about it as far as web security goes, right? Well, not exactly. It's certainly a great start, but there are a few other techniques you need to know before you can truly say you're practicing safe surfing. The rest of this chapter gives you the details.

Creating Secure Passwords

Many websites require a password to access the site's content. For example, on many sites you must log in to access restricted content that's available only to registered users or paid subscribers. On retail sites, you often have an account that's password-protected so that you can place orders and track shipments. Finally, a password is a must for secure sites such as online banking and online investing pages.

Each of these scenarios has a different level of security, but in each case you don't want an unauthorized person to log in using your account. The best way to prevent unauthorized access is to protect your account with a strong password.

Lots of books suggest absurdly fancy password schemes (I've written some of those books myself!), but there are really only three things you need to know to create strong-like-bull passwords:

- **Use passwords that are at least 8 characters long.** Shorter passwords are susceptible to programs that just try every letter combination. You can combine the 26 letters of the alphabet into about 12 million 5-letter word combinations, which is no big deal for a fast program. If you bump things up to 8-letter passwords, however, the total number of combinations rises to 200 *billion*, which would take even the fastest computer quite a while. If you use 12-letter passwords, as many experts recommend, the number of combinations goes beyond mind-boggling: 90 *quadrillion*, or 90,000 trillion!

- **Mix up your character types**. The secret to a strong password is to include characters from the following categories: lowercase letters, uppercase letters, numbers, and symbols. If you include at least one character from three (or even better, all four) of these categories, you're well on your way toward a strong password.

- **Don't be too obvious**. Because forgetting a password is inconvenient, many people use meaningful words or numbers so their password will be easier to remember. Unfortunately, this means that they often use extremely obvious things such as their name, the name of a family member or colleague, their birth date, their Social Security number, or even their site username. Being this obvious is just asking for trouble.

Good to Know!

How will you know whether the password you've come up with fits the definition of strong? One way to find out is to submit the password to an online password complexity checker, such as the Microsoft Password Checker available at https://www.microsoft.com/security/pc-security/password-checker.aspx. Type your password in the Password box, and make sure the Strength indicator says either Strong or BEST.

While we're on the subject of passwords, I should mention that Internet Explorer may from time to time display a message like the one shown in Figure 15.5, asking whether you want it to save a site password that you just entered.

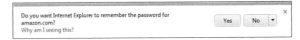

Figure 15.5: Internet Explorer will often ask whether it can save a site password for you.

Should you have Internet Explorer save your password? Sometimes yes and sometimes no is the maddeningly vague answer.

Why would you? When Internet Explorer saves your login data (username and password), it enters that data automatically the next time you access the login portion of the site. This can save a bit of wear and tear on your typing fingers.

Why wouldn't you? Because if someone with malicious (or even just mischievous) intent managed to sit down in front of your computer while it's logged on to Windows, that person could access any website where you've saved the password. Not saving your password ensures that unauthorized users can't access your stuff on that site.

To know which way to go, whenever Internet Explorer asks about saving a password, ask yourself what is the worst thing that could happen if an unauthorized person accesses your account. If you could lose money, have private information exposed, or suffer some other harm, then by all means click **No**; on the other hand, if the risk is minimal (and it often is), then go right ahead and click **Yes**.

Should You Give Out Your Credit Card Information?

As you saw in Chapter 13, if you want to purchase anything online, you pretty much have to use a credit card. However, that brings up a very good question: Just how safe is it to throw your credit card information into cyberspace?

Here's the short answer: it depends. Here's the long answer: it depends on whether the website you're using is secure. How are you supposed to know this? Fortunately, the Internet Explorer window gives you visual cues that tell you whether a particular website is secure. For example, Figure 15.6 shows Internet Explorer displaying a secure web page. Notice how a lock icon appears to the right of the address and that the address of a secure page uses **https** up front rather than **http**. Both of these features tell you that the web page has a security certificate that passed muster with Internet Explorer.

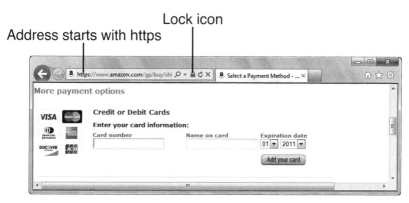

Figure 15.6: If you don't see these features, do not give the site your credit card details.

Deleting Your Browsing History

As you roam the web, Internet Explorer is constantly saving data related to the sites you've seen. This is called your *browsing history*, and saving that data is usually a good thing because it's meant to speed up your surfing. However, it can also be a bad thing because anyone sitting down at your computer can surmise where you've been surfing. If you don't like the sound of that, you can delete your browsing history by following these steps:

1. Click **Tools** (the icon that looks like a gear), then select **Safety, Delete Browsing History** (or press **Ctrl+Shift+Delete**) to display the Delete Browsing History dialog box, shown in Figure 15.7.

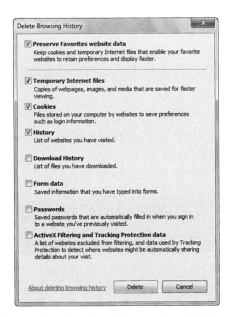

Figure 15.7: Use the Delete Browsing History dialog box to choose what web stuff you want to blow away.

2. If you don't want to save the files associated with sites on your Favorites list, deactivate the **Preserve Favorites website data** check box.

3. Activate the check box beside each type of data you want to smite:

- **Temporary internet files**—these are copies of text, images, media, and other content from the pages you've visited recently. Internet Explorer stores all this data so that the next time you view one of those pages, it can retrieve data from the cache and display the site much more quickly. This is clearly a big-time privacy problem because it means that anyone can examine the cache to learn where you've been surfing.

- **Cookies**—these are small text files that sites store on your computer. Most cookies are benign, but they can be used to track your activities online.

- **History**—this is a list of addresses of the sites you've visited in the past 20 days as well as each of the pages you visited within those sites. Again, this is a major privacy accident just waiting to happen, because anyone sitting at your computer can see exactly where you've been online over the last 20 days.

- **Download History**—this is a list of the files you've downloaded.

- **Form data**—this refers to the AutoComplete feature, which stores the data you type in forms and then uses that saved data to suggest possible matches when you use a similar form in the future. This is definitely handy, but it also means that anyone else who uses your computer can see your previously entered form text.

- **Passwords**—this is another aspect of AutoComplete, and Internet Explorer uses it to save form passwords. As you saw earlier, it's nice and convenient—but it's really just asking for trouble because it means that someone sitting down at your computer can log on to a site (a job made all the easier if you activated the site option to save your username!).

- **ActiveX Filtering and Tracking Protection data**—this is information that Internet Explorer gathers to detect when third-party providers are supplying data to the sites you visit. For more information, see the next section.

4. Click **Delete**.

Browse Privately

Deleting your browsing history is a handy technique for sure, but you have to remember to do it—and it's a distressingly all-or-nothing affair. That is, when you delete form data, passwords, history, cookies, or the cache files, you delete *all* of them (unless you preserve the cookies and cache files for your favorites). This is a problem, because you often only want to remove the data for a single site or a few sites.

Fortunately, Internet Explorer implements a single feature that solves these problems: InPrivate browsing. When you activate this feature, Internet Explorer stops storing private data when you visit websites. It no longer saves temporary internet files, cookies, browsing history, form data, and passwords.

To use InPrivate browsing, click **Tools** and then select **Safety**, **InPrivate Browsing** (or press **Ctrl+Shift+P**). Internet Explorer opens a new browser window, as shown in Figure 15.8. Notice that Internet Explorer reminds you that you're using InPrivate browsing by displaying the InPrivate icon in the address bar.

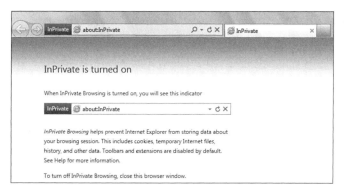

Figure 15.8: When you activate InPrivate browsing, Internet Explorer opens a new window and displays the InPrivate icon in the address bar.

What Can Go Wrong?

When your private session is done, be sure to turn InPrivate browsing off so that Internet Explorer returns to saving your browsing data and you regain use of handy tools such as the History list.

Block Pop-Up Windows

One of the most annoying things on the web are those ubiquitous pop-up windows that infest your screen with advertisements when you visit certain sites. (A variation on the theme is the "pop under," a window that opens "under" your current browser window, so you don't know it's there until you close the window.) And as you saw earlier in this chapter, pop-up windows can also be dangerous because some unscrupulous software makers have figured out ways to use them to install viruses and spyware on your computer without your permission. They're nasty things any way you look at them.

Fortunately, Microsoft has given us a way to stop pop-ups before they start. It's called the Pop-up Blocker, and it looks for pop-ups and prevents them from opening. Follow these steps to use and configure Pop-up Blocker:

1. In Internet Explorer, select **Tools, Internet Options**.
2. Select the **Privacy** tab.
3. Activate the **Turn On Pop-up Blocker** check box (if it isn't on already).
4. Click **Settings** to display the Pop-up Blocker Settings dialog box. You have the following options:
    - **Address of website to allow**   Use this option when you have a site that displays pop-ups you want to see. Enter the address, then click **Add**.
    - **Play a sound when a pop-up is blocked**   When this check box is activated, Internet Explorer plays a brief sound each time it blocks a pop-up. If this gets annoying after a while, deactivate this check box.
    - **Show Information bar when a pop-up is blocked**   When this check box is activated, Internet Explorer displays a yellow bar below the tabs each time it blocks a pop-up—just so you know it's working on your behalf.
    - **Blocking level**   Use this list to choose how aggressive you want Internet Explorer to be with pop-ups. Medium should work fine, but if you still get lots of pop-ups, switch to High.
5. Click **Close**, then click **OK**.

Pop-up Blocker, now on the case, monitors your surfing and steps in front of any pop-up window that tries to disturb your peace. Figure 15.9

shows the Notification bar that pops up (sorry, couldn't resist!) to let you know when a pop-up was thwarted. If you want to see the pop-up anyway, click **Allow once**; if you're okay with this site's pop-ups, click **Options for this site** and then click **Always allow**.

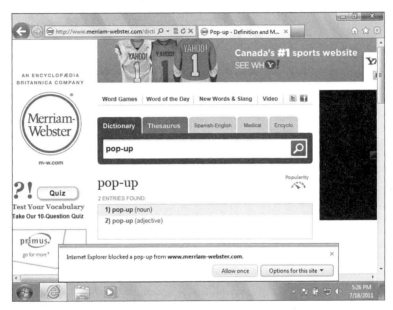

Figure 15.9: When the Pop-up Blocker is active, it displays a Notification bar each time it blocks a pop-up window.

The Least You Need to Know

- Be sure to protect your computer by installing an antivirus program and perhaps a second antispyware program.
- Thumb your nose at suspicious web ads and pop-up windows, and for the latter, make sure you never click anything within the pop-up window.

- Only submit sensitive data (such as your credit card number) to a secure site (that is, one that has a lock icon in the status bar and an address that begins with https).
- If the User Account Control dialog box appears, only give permission if you're sure it's asking about an action you initiated yourself.
- Use secure passwords on websites that require them. This means a password that's at least eight characters, isn't too obvious, and includes characters from at least three out of the following four sets: lowercase letters, uppercase letters, numbers, and symbols.

Keeping Your Email Safe and Sound

Chapter 16

In This Chapter

- Guarding against nasty email viruses
- Putting spam back in the can
- Getting hip to hoaxes and other useless messages
- Blocking annoying or abusive emailers

Email seems like the most innocuous of the internet's many services. After all, what can possibly be bad about exchanging messages with family, friends, and other online citizens? Well, not much, as it turns out, because most email messages are benign. Notice, however, that I said "most," not "all." Unfortunately, some email messages contain threats to your security and privacy. These threats include viruses lurking in file attachments or message code, unsolicited product offers and marketing pitches, and messages that contain bogus or misleading information.

To protect yourself, you need to understand these threats and know what you can do to thwart them. This chapter introduces you to this negative side of the internet's email system and shows you specific steps you can take to keep your email inbox secure and private.

Protecting Yourself Against Email Viruses

Until just a few years ago, the primary method that computer viruses used to propagate themselves was a now-obsolete bit of technology called a "floppy disk." Somewhat similar to a CD or DVD, a floppy disk could store information and you could transfer that data to a computer by inserting the floppy disk into a special drive on the computer. Of course, if the floppy disk happened to contain a virus program, as soon as you inserted the disk the computer would become infected. If you then copied some files to another floppy disk, the virus would surreptitiously add itself to the disk. If you gave the disk to another person, when the recipient inserted the disk, the virus copy would come to life and infect yet another computer.

When the internet became a big deal, viruses adapted (as viruses do) and began propagating either via malicious websites or infected program files downloaded to users' machines (as you saw in the previous chapter).

Over the last few years, however, by far the most productive method for viruses to replicate has been the humble email message. The list of email viruses is a long one, but they all operate more or less the same way: arriving as a message attachment, usually from someone you know. When you open the attachment, the virus infects your computer—and then, without your knowledge, uses your email program and your address book to ship out messages with more copies of itself attached. The nastier versions will also mess with your computer; the soulless beasts may delete data or corrupt files, for example.

Some General Ways to Avoid Email Viruses

You can avoid getting infected by one of these viruses by implementing a few common-sense procedures:

- Never open an attachment that comes from someone you don't know.

- Even if you know the sender, if the attachment isn't something you're expecting, assume the sender's system is infected. Write back and confirm that he or she sent the message.

- Some viruses come packaged as "scripts"—miniature computer programs—that are hidden within messages that use the Rich-Text (HTML) format. This means that the virus can run just by viewing the message! If a message looks suspicious, don't open it: just delete it. (Note that you'll need to turn off the Windows Live Mail reading pane before deleting the message. Otherwise, when you highlight the message, it will appear in the preview pane and set off the virus. Click the **View** tab, click **Reading pane**, and then click **Off**.)

- As I described in Chapter 15, install a top-of-the-line antivirus program—particularly one that checks incoming email.

Windows Live Mail's Antivirus Settings

Besides these general procedures, Windows Live Mail also comes with its own set of virus protection features. Here's how to use them:

1. In Windows Live Mail, select **File**, **Option**, **Safety options**.

2. Display the **Security** tab.

3. In the **Virus Protection** section of the dialog box (see Figure 16.1), you have the following options:

    - **Select the security zone to use.** You use the security zones to determine whether scripts inside HTML-format messages are allowed to run. If you choose internet zone, scripts are allowed to run; if you choose Restricted Sites Zone, scripts are disabled. Restricted Sites Zone is the default setting, and it's the one I highly recommend.

- **Warn me when other applications try to send mail as me.** As I mentioned earlier, it's possible for programs and scripts to send email messages without your knowledge. When you activate this check box, Windows Live Mail displays a warning dialog box when a program or script attempts to send a message behind the scenes.

- **Do not allow attachments to be saved or opened that could potentially be a virus.** When you activate this check box, Windows Live Mail monitors attachments to look for file types that could contain viruses or destructive code. If it detects such a file, it halts the ability to open or save that file, and it displays a note at the top of the message to let you know about the unsafe attachment.

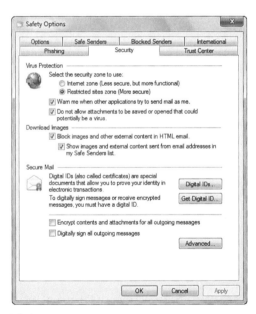

Figure 16.1: Use the Security tab to configure the Windows Live Mail antivirus options.

4. Click **OK**.

5. Select **File**, **Options**, **Mail** to switch to the Options dialog box.

6. Display the **Read** tab.

7. Activate the **Read all messages in plain text** check box.

8. Click **OK**.

Shielding Yourself from the Scourge of Spam

Junk email—which many people refer to as *spam*—refers to unsolicited, commercial email messages that advertise a wide variety of products, from baldness cures to cheap printer cartridges. Junk email product pitches are frustrating to deal with because they clog up your mailbox and you have to waste time deleting them. However, some junk email messages are more than just annoying. For example, many junk messages advertise deals that are simply fraudulent, contain profanity or offensive images, or feature unsavory practices such as linking to adult-oriented sites or to sites that install spyware. So knowing how to minimize the amount of spam you receive is a crucial twenty-first–century survival skill—and this section gives you the full spam scoop.

Definition

Junk email (also known as **spam**) is any unsolicited commercial email message.

Junk ... Spam ... What's Up with These Messages?

Before getting to the anti-spam measures, let's take a second to understand a bit more about these messages. As I mentioned at the top of the section, junk email refers to any email message of a commercial nature that is unsolicited. That is, if you never asked to receive messages from a company, or if you have had no commercial dealings with a company in the recent past, then any commercial messages you receive from that company are classified as junk email. A person or organization that sends such messages is called a *junk emailer* (or, more commonly, a *spammer*). In the United States, by law, unsolicited commercial email must be labeled as such, although few spammers do this.

I should point out here that not all email messages for products or services are spam. If you purchased a product recently, that company may simply be following up with your order. Similarly, if you opted to receive a newsletter or other communications from the company, then the messages are technically not junk email because you asked to have them sent to you.

Still, the amount of junk email sent each day is staggering and has been estimated to comprise between 80 and 90 percent of all daily email traffic. This means that well more than 200 *billion* junk email messages are sent each day, and that number is still growing—although not as quickly as a few years ago, when spam volume was roughly doubling each year.

There are five main types of junk email:

- **Product pitches.** By far the most common type of junk email message is a straightforward advertisement for a commercial product or service. According to spam experts, email advertisements for products (such as fake high-end watches), financial services (particularly for getting out of debt), and health aids (Viagra and related treatments) account for nearly 60 percent of junk email.

- **Offensive messages.** Approximately 20 percent of all junk email messages contain some kind of offensive content. This may include profanity, racist remarks, or other objectionable text. However, most offensive junk email messages are related to adult-oriented websites. This means that the message may contain salacious images, or it may contain one or more links to sites that display such images.

- **Scams.** Many junk email messages are scams that advertise nonexistent products, services, and money-making opportunities. The most common of these is the so-called advance-fee fraud, in which a person is asked for money to help secure the release of, and so earn a percentage of, a much larger sum. These scams often originate in Nigeria, so they are sometimes called 419 scams (because 419 is the section number of the Nigerian penal code that covers this sort of fraudulent behavior). See Chapter 17 for more information.

- **Viruses and spyware.** Many junk email messages do not try to sell you anything at all. Instead, the spam message is really a vehicle for a virus or a spyware program, as described earlier in this chapter.

- **Phishing.** This type of spam message attempts to trick you into supplying confidential or sensitive data. Again, I talk about phishing in more detail in Chapter 17.

How to Avoid Spam

It's clear that spam has become a plague upon the earth. Unless you've done a masterful job at keeping your address secret, you probably receive at least a few spam emails every day—and it's more likely that you receive a few dozen. The bad news is that most experts agree that it's only going to get worse. And why not? Spam is one of the few advertising mediums where the costs are substantially borne by the users, not the advertisers.

The best way to avoid spam is to not get on a spammer's list of addresses in the first place. That's hard to do these days, but there are some steps you can take:

- Never use your actual email address in an online forum or discussion group. The most common method that spammers use to gather addresses is to harvest them from online posts. One common tactic is to alter your email address by adding text that invalidates the address but is still obvious for other people to figure out:

    gclooney@moviestars.remove_this_to_email_me.com

- When you sign up for something online, use a fake address if possible. If you need or want to receive email from the company and so must use your real address, make sure you deselect any options that ask whether you want to receive promotional offers. Alternatively, enter the address from a free web-based account (such as Hotmail) so that any spam you receive will go there instead of to your main address.

- Never open suspected spam messages, because doing so can sometimes notify the spammer that you've opened the message—thus confirming that your address is legit. For the same reason, you should never display a spam message in the Windows Live Mail reading pane. As described earlier, shut off the reading pane before selecting any spam messages that you want to delete.

- Never, I repeat, *never* respond to spam—even to an address within the spam that claims to be a "removal" address. By responding to the spam, all you're doing is proving that your address is legitimate, so you'll just end up getting *more* spam.

Using the Junk Mail Filter to Can Spam

If you do get spam despite these precautions, the good news is that Windows Live Mail comes with a junk email protection feature that can help you cope. Junk email protection is a *spam filter*, which means that it examines each incoming message and applies sophisticated tests to determine whether the message is spam. If the tests determine that the message is probably spam, the email is exiled to a separate Junk Email folder, and you see the message shown in Figure 16.2. It's not perfect (no spam filter is), but with a bit of fine-tuning as described in the next few sections, it can be a very useful anti-spam weapon.

Definition

A **spam filter** is a tool that attempts to separate junk email messages from regular messages and to segregate junk email in a separate folder.

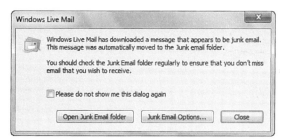

Figure 16.2: Windows Live Mail's spam filter lets you know when it has detected incoming junk messages.

Setting the Junk Email Protection Level

Filtering spam is always a tradeoff between protection and convenience. The stronger the protection you use, the less convenient the filter becomes (and vice-versa). This inverse relationship is caused by a filter phenomenon called the *false positive*. This is a legitimate message that the filter has pegged as spam—and so (in Windows Live Mail's case) moved the message to the Junk Email folder. The stronger the protection level, the more likely it is that false positives will occur, so the more time you must spend checking the Junk Email folder for legitimate messages that need to be rescued. Fortunately, Windows Live Mail gives you several junk email protection levels to choose from, so you can choose a level that gives the blend of protection and convenience that suits you.

To set the junk email protection level in Windows Live Mail, select **File**, **Option**, **Safety options**. Windows Live Mail displays the Safety Options dialog box, and you should see the Options tab (see Figure 16.3) automatically.

If you have Windows Vista and you're using Windows Mail, select **Tools, Junk Email Options**. If you have Windows XP and are using Outlook Express, then I regret to inform you that no spam filter is available. However, Windows Live Mail does run on Windows XP (with Service Pack 2 or later installed), so consider installing that program.

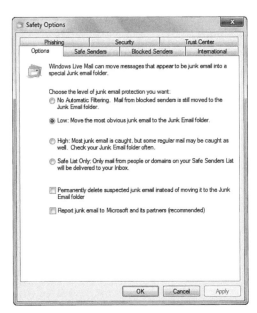

Figure 16.3: Use the Options tab to configure the Windows Live Mail spam filter.

The Options tab gives you four choices for the junk email protection level:

- **No Automatic Filtering** This option turns off the spam filter. I don't recommend this option—not even a little.

- **Low** This is the default protection level, and it's designed to move only messages with obvious spam content to the Junk Email folder. This is a good level to start with—particularly if you get only a few spams a day—because it catches most spam and has only a minimal risk of false positives.

- **High** This level handles spam aggressively and only rarely misses a junk message. On the downside, the High level also catches the occasional legitimate message in its nets, so you need to check the Junk Email folder regularly to look for false positives. Use this level if you get a lot of spam—a few dozen messages or more each day.

By the Way

If you get a false positive in your Junk Email folder, either drag the message back to your Inbox folder, or click the message, click the **Home** tab, and then click the top half of the **Not junk** button (the green check mark).

- **Safe List Only** This level treats all incoming messages as spam except for those messages that come from people or domains in your Safe Senders list (see "Specifying Safe Senders" later in the chapter). Use this level if your spam problem is out of control (100 or more spam messages each day) and if most of your non-spam email comes from people you know or from mailing lists you subscribe to.

If you hate spam so much that you never want to even *see* it, much less deal with it, activate the **Permanently delete suspected junk email instead of moving it to the Junk Email folder** check box.

> **What Can Go Wrong?**
>
> Spam is so hair-pullingly frustrating that you may be tempted to activate the **Permanently delete suspected junk email instead of moving it to the Junk Email folder** check box out of sheer spite. I don't recommend this, however. The danger of false positives is just too great, even with the Low level—and it's not worth missing a crucial message.

Identifying Hoaxes and Other Annoyances

It's a rare internet user who hasn't received an email message along the following lines:

> Subject: FW: Must Read!!!! Bill Gates (fwd)
>
> Hello everybody, My name is Bill Gates. I have just written up an email tracing program that traces everyone to whom this message is forwarded to.
>
> I am experimenting with this and I need your help. Forward this to everyone you know and if it reaches 1000 people everyone on the list will receive $1000 at my expense. Enjoy.
>
> Your friend,
>
> Bill Gates

Heeding the last sentence, less-savvy users will most likely have forwarded this warning to a few dozen friends, relatives, and colleagues. There's only one problem: this message is, of course, a hoax. There is no "tracing program," and there is no $1,000 pot of gold at the end of the email rainbow.

This email hoax is part of the general category of email chain letters. Some of these messages claim to be from malicious hackers who will do something nasty to your computer if you don't forward the message to 10 of your friends.

Unfortunately, bogus offers and chain letters aren't the only kind of email hoax going around. Another popular type is the virus hoax, where the message warns you about an email that contains a virus that will wreck your hard drive (or perform some other unpleasant chore). They usually warn you to watch out for a specific subject line, such as "Good Times" (this is the oldest such hoax; it has been around since about 1994), "Win a Holiday," "Penpal Greetings," and many more.

The ironic thing about all this is that these messages end up as a kind of virus themselves. With thousands of people naively forwarding tens of thousands of copies of the message all over the internet, they end up wasting bandwidth and wasting the time of those people who must refute their claims.

I receive many of these hoaxes forwarded from well-meaning readers. Fortunately, the internet offers many sources of information on these hoaxes, so people learn about them pretty fast. If you receive a virus warning or other email that seems legitimate, you can check it out using any of the following sites:

- www.snopes.com
- http://urbanlegends.about.com/
- www.scambusters.org

> **By the Way**
>
> If you do discover that a message is actually a hoax, be sure to send a message to the original sender to let her know. That way, she'll know not to repeat her mistake!

Identifying Good Guys and Bad Guys

As a final method of configuring your email for more security, you can add people to two different lists maintained by Windows Live Mail: the Safe Senders list of people from whom you want to receive messages and the Blocked Senders list of people from whom you do not want to receive mail.

Specifying Safe Senders

If you use the Low or High Junk Email protection level, you can reduce the number of false positives by letting Windows Live Mail know about the people or institutions that regularly send you mail. By designating these addresses as Safe Senders, you tell Windows Live Mail to automatically leave their incoming messages in your Inbox and never to redirect them to the Junk Email folder. And certainly, if you use the Safe Lists Only protection level, you must specify some Safe Senders—because Windows Live Mail treats everyone else as a spammer!

Your Safe Senders list can consist of three types of addresses:

- **Individual email addresses of the form** *someone@somewhere.com*. All messages from these individual addresses will not be treated as spam.

- **Domain names of the form** *@somewhere.com*. All messages from any address within that domain will not be treated as spam.

- **Your Contacts list.** This means that Windows Live Mail treats everyone in your Contacts list as a Safe Sender, which makes sense because you're unlikely to be spammed by someone you know. This setting is turned on by default in Windows Live Mail.

You can specify a Safe Sender either by entering the address by hand (using the Safe Senders tab in the Safety Options dialog box) or by using an existing message from the sender (click the message you want to work with, click the **Home** tab, click the bottom half of the **Junk** button, and then select either **Add sender to safe sender list** or **Add sender's domain to safe sender list**).

In Windows Vista, if you're using Windows Mail, select **Tools**, **Junk Email Options**, and then click the **Safe Senders** tab. In Windows XP, Outlook Express doesn't offer a Safe Senders list. (Although again, you can install Windows Live Mail if you'd like to use this feature.)

Blocking Senders

If you notice that a particular address is the source of much spam or other annoying email, the easiest way to block the spam is to block all incoming messages from that address. You can do this by using the Blocked Senders list, which watches for messages from a specific address and relegates them to the Junk Email folder.

As with Safe Senders, you can specify a Blocked Sender either by entering the address by hand (using the Blocked Senders tab in the Safety Options dialog box) or by using an existing message from the sender (click the message you want to work with, click the **Home** tab, click the bottom half of the **Junk** button, and then select either **Add sender to blocked sender list** or **Add sender's domain to blocked sender list**).

If you're a Windows Vista user and you're doing the email thing with Windows Mail, click the message, select **Message**, **Junk Email**, and then select either **Add Sender to Blocked Senders List** or **Add Sender's Domain to Blocked Senders List**. If you're a Windows XP user and you email with Outlook Express, click the message, select **Message**, **Block Sender**, and then click **Yes** to remove the person's messages.

The Least You Need to Know

- To guard against email-borne viruses, never open attachments that come from strangers, and double-check with friends before opening unexpected attachments they send your way.
- To cut down on the spam you receive, don't use your real address in a newsgroup; use a fake address whenever possible when signing up for things online; and never respond to spam or even open suspected spam messages.
- To ensure that a person's message doesn't get flagged as spam, click a message from that person, click the **Home** tab, click the bottom half of the **Junk** button, and then select **Add sender to safe sender list**.
- To block a person from sending you email, click a message from that person, click the **Home** tab, click the bottom half of the **Junk** button, and then select **Add sender to blocked sender list**.

Avoiding Scams

Chapter
17

In This Chapter

- Foiling phishing
- Keeping your identity safe
- Watching out for online fraud
- Guarding against scams when shopping online

In the eighteenth century, a European nobleman named Wolfgang von Kempelen built a chess-playing "machine" that not only "knew" how to play the game but also handily beat anyone who played against it. "The Turk," as it was nicknamed, was in reality an elaborate hoax, and its secret was the live human hidden inside the machine.

In the nineteenth century, certain quacks would set up shop in fairs and towns to sell supposedly medicinal potions. To demonstrate the healing powers of these "remedies," a young boy (secretly the charlatan's assistant) would swallow a toad, which in those days was thought to be poisonous. The lad would duly keel over, but a quick sip of the medicine would have him back on his feet.

In the twentieth century, the streets of any major city were home to various flimflam artists hawking bamboozlements such as the shell game, three-card monte, and five-cup turnover as well as larger and more complex bits of chicanery such as Ponzi schemes and pyramid schemes.

This short history lesson is to remind you that con artists, impostors, and swindlers have been around for a long time. No one should be surprised that here in the twenty-first century, the world's scammers and shysters have moved their nefarious trades online—where they can take advantage of the speed and anonymity that the web affords. It's an unfortunate fact of life that these digital bilkers and bunco artists like to prey on older folks, so all the more reason to arm yourself with some knowledge about the scams they try to pull and how to avoid them. This chapter provides you with the real deal.

Understanding Phishing Scams

Phishing refers to creating a replica of an existing web page or using false emails to fool you into submitting personal information, financial data, or a password. It's a whimsical word for a serious bit of business, but the term comes from the fact that internet scammers are using increasingly sophisticated lures as they "fish" for your sensitive data.

Definition

Phishing is a scam that uses bogus email messages and websites to fool you into submitting sensitive or private data, financial information, or a password.

The most common ploy is to copy the web page code from a major site—such as America Online or eBay—and use that code to set up a replica page that appears to be part of the company's site. You receive a fake email with a link to this page, which solicits your credit card data or password. When you submit the form, it sends the data to the scammer while leaving you on an actual page from the company's site so you don't suspect a thing.

Phishing Email Messages

A phishing message is a junk email message that appears to come from a legitimate organization, such as a bank, a major retailer, or an internet service provider. The message will ask you to update your information or warn you that your account is about to expire. In most cases, the message offers a link to a bogus website that tries to fool you into revealing sensitive or private data.

Never trust any email message or website that asks you to update or confirm sensitive data, such as your bank account number, credit card information, Social Security number, or account password. It's important to remember that no legitimate company or organization will ever contact you via email to update or confirm such information online.

It's easy for a phishing scammer to craft an email message that looks like it came from a legitimate organization. However, there are ways to recognize a phishing message:

- If the message is addressed to an individual but you see something like, "Undisclosed recipients" in the To line, then something's fishy (or should I say *phishy*?) right off the bat.

- The message appears to come from a major corporation or organization, but the text contains numerous spelling and grammatical errors—or even misspells the name of the company!

- Position the mouse pointer over any links in the message and examine the address that appears in the status bar. If the address is clearly one that is not associated with the company, as shown in Figure 17.1, then the message is almost certainly a phishing attempt.

Good to Know!

When examining an email link, be particularly on the lookout for addresses that contain a bunch of numbers, such as the http://203.208.24.158 that begins the address shown in Figure 17.1. In the context of the seemingly legitimate email message, these kinds of addresses are always bogus and highly suspicious.

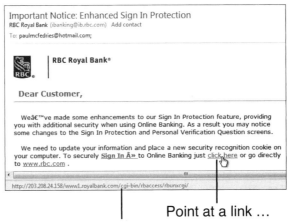

Point at a link …

… and see whether the address looks suspicious (like this one).

Figure 17.1: One way to recognize a phishing message is to position the mouse pointer over a link and then look for a bogus address in the status bar.

If you use Windows Vista and its Windows Mail program, an anti-phishing feature is available. Select **Tools, Junk Email Options**, click the **Phishing** tab, and then activate the **Protect my Inbox from messages with potential Phishing links** check box. Windows XP's Outlook Express program doesn't offer any anti-phishing tools.

Windows Live Mail's Anti-Phishing Tools

Windows Live Mail comes with an anti-phishing feature that can examine received messages for signs of possible phishing activity. You should make sure that this feature is turned on by following these steps:

1. Select **File, Options, Safety options** to open the Safety Options dialog box.

2. Select the **Phishing tab**.

3. Activate the **Protect my Inbox from messages with potential Phishing links**, as shown in Figure 17.2.

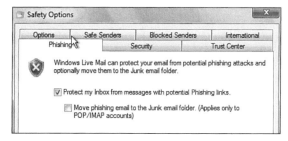

Figure 17.2: Make sure that Windows Live Mail's anti-phishing filter is on the job.

4. To avoid phishing messages stinking up your Inbox, you should also activate the **Move phishing email to the Junk email folder** check box.

5. Click **OK**.

> **Good to Know!**
>
> It's important to bear in mind that some scammers also use phone phishing, where they ask you to call a telephone number to update your data.

With the phishing filter turned on, Windows Live Mail examines each incoming message for telltale phishing characteristics. If Windows Live Mail comes across such a message, it displays the message in red. If you open the message, you see a notice that Windows Live Mail believes the message to be suspicious and that it has blocked any images and links contained in the message (see Figure 17.3). Unless you are sure the message is legitimate, you should click **Delete** to remove the message.

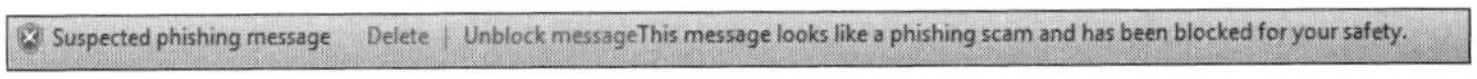

Figure 17.3: Windows Live Mail warns you if it detects a message with telltale phishing characteristics.

Phishing Websites

A phishing page looks identical to a legitimate page from the company because the phisher has simply copied the underlying source code from the original page. However, no spoof page can be a perfect replica of the original. Here are four things to look for:

- **Weirdness in the address** A legitimate page will have the correct domain—such as aol.com or ebay.com—while a spoofed page will have only something similar, such as aol.whatever.com or blah.com/ebay.

- **Weirdness in the addresses associated with page links** Most links on the page probably point to legitimate pages on the original site. However, there may be some links that point to pages on the phisher's site.

- **Text or images that aren't associated with the trustworthy site** Many phishing sites are housed on free web-hosting services. However, many of these services place an advertisement on each page, so look for an ad or other content from the hosting provider.

- **No lock icon** A legitimate site would only transmit sensitive financial data using a secure connection, which Internet Explorer indicates by placing a lock icon in the Address box, as described in Chapter 15. If you don't see the lock icon with a page that asks for financial data, then the page is almost certainly a spoof.

Internet Explorer's Anti-Phishing Tools

If you watch for these things, you'll probably never be fooled into giving up sensitive data to a phisher. However, phishing attacks are becoming legion, so we need all the help we can get. To that end, Internet Explorer comes with a tool called the SmartScreen Filter. This filter alerts you to potential phishing scams by doing two things each time you visit a site:

- Analyzing the site content to look for known phishing techniques
- Checking to see whether the site is listed in a global database of known phishing sites

Phishing has become such a problem that Internet Explorer doesn't even bother to ask you whether you want to use the SmartScreen Filter; it just turns it on by default. To make sure the SmartScreen Filter is on, click **Tools** (the gear icon), and then click **Safety**. If you see a command named **Turn off SmartScreen Filter**, that means the filter is activated and you can move on with your life. On the other hand, if you see the **Turn on SmartScreen Filter** command, click it. In the Microsoft SmartScreen Filter dialog box that displays, make sure the **Turn on SmartScreen Filter** option is activated, then click **OK**.

Here's how the SmartScreen Filter works:

- If you come upon a site that Internet Explorer knows is a phishing scam, it changes the background color of the Address bar to red and displays an Unsafe Website message in the Security Report area (just to the right of the address; see Figure 17.4). It also blocks navigation to the site by displaying a separate page that tells you the site is a known phishing scam.

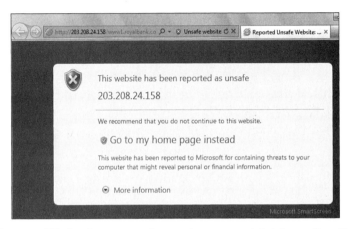

Figure 17.4: If you surf to a known phishing site, the SmartScreen Filter displays this warning and blocks access to the site.

- If you come upon a site that Internet Explorer thinks is a potential phishing scam, it changes the background color of the Address bar to yellow and displays a Suspicious Website message in the Security Report area.

For the latter, click the Suspicious Website text and Internet Explorer displays a security report with a link that enables you to report the site. If you're sure this is a scam site, be sure to report it to help improve the database of phishing sites and prevent others from giving up sensitive data.

Preventing Identity Theft

"Identity theft" sounds like a plot device straight out of a bad B movie, but it's actually a serious crime that the United States Federal Trade Commission (FTC) estimates affects up to nine million people each year. *Identity theft* is the unauthorized and unlawful use of information that personally identifies a person, including that person's name, address, Social Security number, and credit card data.

> **Definition**
>
> **Identity theft** is the illegal use of data that personally identifies a person and enables the thief to commit fraud in that person's name.

Identity thieves use that information to commit fraud in the victim's name, and these fraudulent activities can take many forms:

- Opening new accounts in the victim's name, including bank accounts, credit cards, phone lines, and utilities. They don't pay the bills owing on these accounts, of course, and the delinquent payments appear on the victim's credit report.

- Running up charges on your existing accounts. Many identity thieves also change the account's billing address so the victim doesn't see the bogus charges until it's way too late.

- Defrauding banks, businesses, and the government, including taking out loans, renting apartments or houses, getting jobs, getting driver's licenses, receiving government benefits, and even filing tax returns—all in the victim's name.

Clearly, identity theft is a serious bit of business—and it's important to take steps to prevent your identity from falling into the wrong hands.

We're talking here about staying safe online, but first you should know that there are some easy steps you can take offline to help prevent identity theft. These include shredding unneeded financial documents and papers that contain personal information; keeping a close eye on your finances to look for suspicious activity, such as credit card charges for goods or services you didn't purchase; obtaining a copy of your credit report and scouring it for unusual activities or inaccurate information; and watching out for missed bills and account statements (identity thieves often use change-of-address forms to divert bills and statements to a different address).

By the Way

To get a free copy of your credit report, contact one of the nationwide credit report firms: Equifax (www.equifax.com), Experian (www.experian.com), or TransUnion (www.transunion.com).

ID thieves use plenty of offline methods to gather personal information (such as going through your trash or stealing your wallet or purse), but these days much of the action is online. Here are a few things you can do to help keep your information safe and out of the grubby paws of identity thieves:

- Never give out your Social Security number (or the equivalent in your country, such as the Social Insurance Number in Canada). Yes, it uniquely identifies you, but any reputable site will take some other form of ID. If a site insists, take your business elsewhere.

- Only give your name, address, and phone number to reputable sites or to sites that you know are legit. The same goes for information about your relatives, including personal data for your spouse, siblings, children, and grandchildren.

- Never give out data related to your vehicle, including its make and model, license plate number, vehicle identification number (VIN), your insurance company and account details, loan information, and your driver's license number.

- Learn to recognize phishing email messages and websites, as described earlier in this chapter, because phishing is now a very common method that identity thieves use to gather personal data.

- Use strong passwords for all websites and email accounts, as described in Chapter 15. Those few letters, numbers, and symbols are often the only things that stand between you and a would-be thief, so it's not hyperbole to say that your financial health and personal reputation depend on them.

- Just say "No" when a website asks you to provide your credit history or credit rating. No site needs to know this stuff.

> **What Can Go Wrong?**
>
> There are plenty of websites that purport to offer free credit ratings and reports. Don't believe them! These sites are just fronts for scammers trying to extract your credit history and other personal data.

Protecting Yourself from "419" Scams

Many junk email messages are scams that advertise nonexistent products, services, and money-making opportunities. The most common of these is the so-called *advance fee fraud*, in which a person is asked for money to help secure the release of a much larger sum with the promise of sharing the riches in return for that help. These scams often originate in Nigeria, so they're sometimes called *Nigerian letter scams* or *419 scams*, because 419 is the section number of the Nigerian penal code that covers this sort of fraudulent behavior.

419 scams almost always originate as email messages, and the details vary but the overall story is the same:

- The writer has access to lots of money—typically, several million dollars. In most of these scams, the writer needs to shield the money from a corrupt government, has won a lottery or inheritance, needs help converting the currency, or wants to give the money to charity.

- The writer creates an impressively detailed persona and situation to sound plausible (see Figure 17.5).

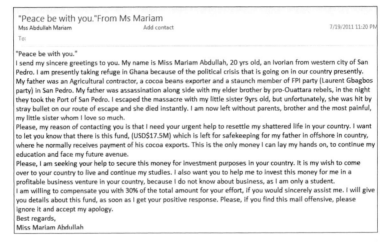

Figure 17.5: A typical 419 scam email message.

- For arcane and complex reasons, the writer needs help getting the money out of his home country.

- You, as a person of outstanding character and honesty, are just the person to help.

Of course, "helping" means first sending some cash to cover "transfer" fees or "account" fees. Then, an even larger sum is required to pay for a lawyer or an accountant. Then, hundreds of dollars are needed for bribing certain government or law-enforcement officials. Finally, thousands of dollars are requested for airfare or other transportation costs. The result: you're out a few thousand dollars or more, and you never hear from the scammer again.

If you receive an apparently all-too-sincere email from a polite and well-connected foreigner who needs to liberate millions of dollars and is offering you a large chunk of that fortune to help, there's only one thing you should do: hit the Delete key!

Preventing Fraud When Shopping Online

You learned all kinds of useful things about shopping-'til-you-drop on the web back in Chapter 13. However, although I spent a good deal of time talking about the positive aspects of online purchasing, I didn't dwell all that much on the negative side—particularly the 800-pound gorilla in the online shopping mall: fraud. Yes, unfortunately there are online equivalents of butchers with their thumbs on the scale and bait-and-switch retailers who advertise one thing and try to sell you another.

To help you see through these charlatans and double-dealers, the next couple sections offer some advice for avoiding scams with online shopping and auction sites.

General Considerations

When it comes to avoiding online shopping fraudsters, the number one rule is a simple one: if a price seems too good to be true, it almost certainly is. Yes, some retailers occasionally offer a product as a *loss leader*—a price that's substantially lower than their competitors as a way of tempting you to buy something and thus establish a relationship with the store. (After you purchase at least one thing from a store, you're more likely to go back—particularly if the experience was a positive one.) However, it's also entirely possible for some of the shadier outfits to offer super-low prices on returned or refurbished products without telling you what you're getting. Unless you know the store is reputable, assume really low prices are bogus and move on to the next online store.

Following on from that last point, note that a really cheap price may be the *net* price you pay after processing a mail-in rebate. Obviously, you'll pay a higher price up front, but some retailers don't tell you that—or they hide the fact in small print somewhere. Also, beware of extra "handling" charges and other fees that the retailer might try to tack on. Before committing to the sale, always give the invoice a thorough going-over so you know exactly what you're paying.

Indeed, most good online vendors will give you a chance during checkout to enter your ZIP code or postal code so you can see exactly what your shipping charges will be (see Figure 17.6). Because the cost of shipping can often be extravagant, whenever possible you should find out the cost in advance before completing the sale.

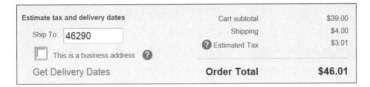

Figure 17.6: If offered, be sure to enter your ZIP or postal code to see the exact shipping charges on your order.

The Best Way to Pay

When it comes time to pay, some retailers allow you to mail a check or money order and will ship the order when they receive payment. You should avoid these payment options like the plague, however, because if something goes wrong (for example, the product never shows up), getting your money back could be a challenge. If you pay by credit card, however, you always have the option of charging back the cost to the vendor.

> **What Can Go Wrong?**
>
> Watch out for online retailers who charge some kind of extra fee (usually a percentage of the product price) for accepting credit card payments. This is almost always a sign of a shady dealer who's either trying to squeeze an extra few percentage points out of you or is trying to discourage you from using a credit card.

A credit card is the way to go. However, you should only enter your credit card data in a payment window that is secure. See Chapter 15 for the details, but remember to look for Internet Explorer's lock icon and an address that starts with "https" instead of "http." Also, many retailers offer the option of saving your credit card data. It's awfully tempting not to have to type all those numbers every time you purchase something from a site, but don't do it. The most common method that online crooks use to steal credit card information is to break in to retailer computer systems and pilfer all the saved credit card data.

If you really want to avoid entering your credit card data, use PayPal if the retailer offers it as a payment option (see Figure 17.7). Currently owned by eBay, PayPal is an online payment service that enables you to buy online without exposing your credit card data to the retailer. You sign up for a PayPal account at www.paypal.com and provide them with your credit card, debit card, or bank account information. (It's all super-secure, and everything is verified before your account goes online.) When you buy something online with a PayPal-friendly retailer, that retailer tells PayPal the cost of the sale and PayPal charges it to your credit card, debit card, or bank account—then passes along the money to the retailer. The retailer never sees your financial data, so you never have to worry about that data being stolen or accidentally exposed.

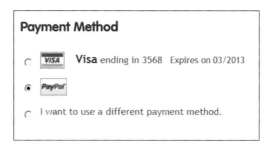

Figure 17.7: Sign up with super-safe PayPal, then look for online retailers who offer a PayPal payment option to avoid exposing your credit card data.

Avoiding Online Auction Fraud

Online auctions can be lots of fun, and they're a great way to save tons of money on things you need (or even things you don't). However, although professional retailers do have a presence on the major online auction sites (such as eBay), most of the time you'll be dealing with individuals much like you who are just looking to unload some of their stuff.

But you can also come across lots of people who are only too happy to take advantage of the anonymity inherent in online transactions to pull a fast one or two on unsuspecting buyers.

All well-run auction sites allow users to rate the people they deal with on the site. If a seller offers timely delivery of the exact products advertised, then that person would tend to garner a high rating while a shady dealer who is slow on delivery or doesn't send the product at all would tend to generate low ratings.

When you're deciding whether to bid on an item, first check the rating of the seller and avoid any auctions run by low-rated sellers. Even if the seller appears to be okay, you should also check the rating of the first people to bid on the item or the people with the most recent bids. Some scammers work with teams who artificially bid up the price of an item, so low-rated bidders could be a sign that this so-called *shilling* (also called *shill bidding*) is going on.

> **What Can Go Wrong?**
>
> If you're selling an item, keep an eye out for *bid shielding*. This is the practice of placing a low bid in an online auction and having a second person enter a bid that is high enough to discourage other bidders. At the last second, the high bid is retracted and the low bid wins.

Also, beware of any auction seller who contacts you outside the auction. For example, the seller may say that the person who won the bid has reneged, so he or she offers the item to you directly. This is an auction no-no, because most reputable auction sites offer some fraud protection as long as you make the purchase within an auction. Once you make the transaction outside an auction, you lose that protection. The most likely result here is that the seller will take your money and you'll never see the item.

For more expensive items, you should contact the seller and ask for proof of ownership (for example, a vehicle title or registration) or proof of possession (for example, a photo where you request the specific shot, which could be of a specific part of the item or taken from a unique angle).

A credit card is the best way to pay for something you buy at an online auction, because if the item never shows up or if the seller sends you an item that is damaged or inferior to the one advertised, then you can ask the credit card company to charge back the payment. However, you *really* don't want to expose your credit card data in an online auction setting. This is where PayPal (which I discussed in the previous section) is perfect, because the seller gets paid quickly and you keep your financial information safe.

Check Overpayment Scams

The *check overpayment scam* (also known as the *wire-transfer scam*) qualifies as an oldie but goodie. You sell something online using an auction site such as eBay (www.ebay.com) or a classified site such as Craigslist (www.craigslist.org), and let's say the selling price was $100. Nice! However, the buyer sends you a check for $1,000 and claims it was an accidental slip of the pen. No matter, he or she says, just go ahead and cash the check and then wire the $900 difference.

I think you may guess where this sad story ends up: you end up with a bounced check, and the buyer ends up with $900 cash—*and* the item you sold him or her!

The lesson: make sure a check clears your bank before wiring an overpayment back to the buyer (and before shipping the item to the buyer).

Bogus Health Products

If I had a dollar for every email or website ad I've seen marketing a miracle cure "that doctors don't want you to know about" or a diet secret "that melts away fat," then I surely wouldn't spend those thousands of dollars on any of these bogus products!

Earlier, I mentioned that the first rule for avoiding online shopping fraud is as follows: if a price seems too good to be true, it almost certainly is. A corollary to that is: if a marketing pitch makes claims for a product that sound too good to be true, they almost certainly are.

We're all concerned about our health, particularly as we get older, so it will come as no surprise that most of the bogus products are health-related: disease cures, weight-loss regimes, anti-aging products, hair-loss restoration ointments … you name it. No reputable doctor or company would advertise products this way, so any such ad you see almost certainly comes from someone disreputable whose only goal is to exchange a worthless product for your hard-earned cash. If you think there's a tiny chance that a health product may live up to its claims, ask your doctor before plunking down any cash.

> **What Can Go Wrong?**
>
> If you come across a website that asks you to fill in a questionnaire regarding your health, say "No thanks" and move on to another site. These questionnaires are only designed to elicit any health problems or symptoms you may be experiencing, so the site can then send you marketing pitches for products that just happen to "alleviate" those symptoms.

Also, beware the many fake online pharmacies offering cheap prescription drugs. How can you tell which ones are fake? They're the ones that claim to offer prescription drugs, but they don't ask you for a prescription! Also, you won't find any contact details—no street address and no phone number—anywhere on the site. The absence of contact details is a sure sign of a bogus or shady online retail operation, regardless of the products they're selling.

"Free" Offers That Aren't So Free

Economists used to tell us that there's no such thing as a free lunch. Meals still aren't usually free, but there's plenty of free stuff floating around the internet. (Technically, you're still "paying" for this free content through your ISP fees, by having to look at ads on the site and so on, but I digress.) However, on the web there's free, and then there's "free."

By that I mean that with some of the web's apparently free lunches, not only do you have to pay the tab but you also have to pay for the privilege of eating—plus you often give your credit card information to a fraud artist as dessert.

These bogus free offers litter the web. Through emails or website ads, they offer free access to sites that normally require payment, free music downloads, free vacations, free iPods, free product trials, free prizes for being "the 10,000 visitor!" (see Figure 17.8), and so on.

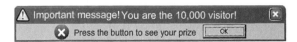

Figure 17.8: An example of an internet come-on that you should studiously ignore.

To confuse matters, some legitimate companies offer free stuff, so how do you tell the legit operators from the shysters? Here are some things to look for:

- The ad contains misspellings or grammatical errors.
- Clicking a link in the ad just leads to another ad.
- The company requires a fee up front to claim your prize.
- The company asks for your credit card or bank data.
- The company tries to convince you to instead purchase a "deluxe" or "advanced" version of the free product.

If you see any of these things, move on to a different message or site—and be thankful that yet another "free" offer hasn't cost you big bucks.

The Least You Need to Know

- Phishing is a scam that uses bogus email messages and websites to fool you into submitting sensitive or private data, financial information, or a password.
- To recognize a phishing email, look for typos in the text and links that aren't associated with the company.
- Identity theft is the illegal use of data that personally identifies a person and enables the thief to commit fraud in that person's name.
- Avoid identity theft by never giving out your Social Security number, by offering personal data only to reputable sites, and by protecting your accounts with strong passwords.
- When shopping online, remember that if a deal appears too good to be true, it almost always is.

Glossary

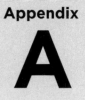

Appendix A

419 scam   A fraud where a scammer asks you for money to help secure the release of a larger sum, with the promise of sharing the riches in return for your help.

ADSL   Broadband internet access offered by the telephone company (short for Asymmetric Digital Subscriber Line).

antispyware program   A software program that blocks or eradicates spyware.

antivirus program   A software program that blocks or eradicates computer viruses.

attachment   A file, such as a photo or text document, that accompanies an email message.

Bcc   A blind courtesy (or carbon) copy email message. These are copies of the message that get sent to other people, but their addresses aren't shown to the other recipients. *See also* Cc.

bid shielding   The practice of placing a low bid in an online auction and having a second person enter a bid that is high enough to discourage other bidders. At the last second, the high bid is retracted and the low bid wins.

bit   Short for "binary digit"; represents the most basic unit of computer information.

boot To start your computer.

bps Stands for bits per second; used to measure the speed at which the modem spews data through a phone line.

broadband High-speed internet access.

broadband modem A device that your computer connects to for high-speed internet access.

browser *See* web browser.

burn To copy a selection of files to a recordable CD or DVD using a CD/DVD burner.

byte Eight bits strung together, which represents a single character of data.

caption bar *See* title bar.

Cc A courtesy (or carbon) copy. These are copies of an email message that get sent to other people. *See also* Bcc.

CD A compact disc, which is a data storage medium that looks much like a music CD.

CD/DVD burner A type of CD/DVD drive that enables you to record data to a CD or DVD.

CD/DVD drive A disc drive that contains a slot or tray designed to read CDs or DVDs.

central processing unit (CPU) The device that coordinates everything that happens inside your computer.

check box A dialog box control that toggles a setting on and off.

check overpayment scam When a buyer "accidentally" sends you a check for an amount larger than the selling price and asks you to cash the check and return the difference.

click To press and immediately release the left mouse button.

clipboard An area of your computer's memory that Windows uses to store the data that you cut or copy from a document.

command A pull-down menu item that initiates some kind of action within a program.

command button A dialog box control that executes a command.

computer case The main box that houses the internal components that enable the computer to run, as well as the external ports that enable you to attach devices to the computer.

control A dialog box feature that you use to manipulate a particular setting.

cookie A small text file that a website adds to your computer to store things like your shopping cart contents and your site preferences.

coupon code A value that you enter when purchasing something online to receive a discount or some other special deal.

CPU *See* central processing unit.

cropping When editing a digital photo, specifying a rectangular area that you want to keep while discarding everything outside the rectangle.

desktop The part of the Windows screen above the taskbar. It's called a "desktop" because it's where your documents and tools appear.

desktop case A style of computer case that's short with a relatively wide base. *See also* tower case.

dial-up A connection to a network (or an internet service provider) that occurs via a modem over a phone line.

dialog box A small window that a program uses to prompt you for more information or to display a message.

digital camera A film camera–like device that takes pictures of the outside world and stores them digitally for later downloading to a hard disk.

document A file that you created yourself or that someone else created and sent to you.

document window A window within a program window that contains a document.

domain name The internet location of a particular website.

double-click To quickly press and release the left mouse button *twice* in succession.

download To receive data from a remote computer. *See also* upload.

download speed The rate at which your ISP sends data from the internet to your computer, which is usually faster than upload speed.

drag To move an object using your mouse by placing the mouse pointer over the object, holding down a mouse button (usually the left button), and then moving the mouse.

drop To use your mouse to place an object in a new location; releasing the mouse button after you have dragged the object to its new home.

drop-down list box A list box that displays only the selected item.

DSL *See* ADSL.

DVD A digital video disc, which is a data storage medium similar to a CD except that it can store much more data.

e-zine An online magazine with no print equivalent.

ergonomics A set of principles and practices for setting up a computer work area to help to maximize comfort and safety.

false positive A regular email message that a spam filter has marked as junk email.

favorite A web page name and address saved within Internet Explorer for easy recall down the road.

flash drive A small USB device used for storing files.

focus The dialog box control that you are currently working with.

folder A storage location for files and other folders (subfolders).

fridge Googling Running an internet search for a recipe based on some or all of the ingredients in your refrigerator.

friend A person with whom you are connected on Facebook; to create a connection with someone on Facebook.

function key A key that begins with the letter F—such as F1 and F2—that performs a specific function.

gigabyte About 1,000 megabytes. Those in-the-know usually abbreviate this as "GB" when writing and as "gig" when speaking. *See also* byte, kilobyte, and megabyte.

group coupon An online deal that only comes into effect if a specified minimum number of people sign up to make the purchase.

hard drive The main storage area inside your computer.

hardware The physical components that make up your system.

icon A small picture that represents something on your computer.

identity theft The illegal use of data that personally identifies a person and enables the thief to commit fraud in that person's name.

IMAP (Internet Message Access Protocol) A set of technologies that enable you to work with email messages that are stored on a remote mail server.

insertion point cursor The blinking vertical bar you see inside a text box or in a word-processing application, such as WordPad. It indicates where the next character you type will appear.

install To add a program to your computer.

internet service provider (ISP) A company that takes your money in exchange for an internet account, which is what you need to get online.

ISP *See* internet service provider.

junk email Unsolicited, commercial email messages.

key combination A keyboard technique where you hold down one key and then press another key (or possibly two other keys).

keyboard A typewriter-like device that you use to enter information.

kilobyte Approximately 1,000 bytes. To be hip, always abbreviate this to "K" or "KB." *See also* megabyte and gigabyte.

library A special type of folder designed to store specific kinds of files, such as documents or pictures.

link On a web page, a chunk of text or an image that, when clicked, takes you to another website.

list box A dialog box control that displays a list of items where you click the item you want to use.

log on To provide your internet service provider with your username and password.

mail server A computer that your ISP uses to store and send your email messages. *See also* server.

mapping site A website that enables you to view and manipulate maps.

media player A device such as an iPod or iPad that plays music, movies, and videos.

megabyte   Approximately 1,000 kilobytes or 1,000,000 bytes. The experts write this as "M" or "MB" and pronounce it "meg." *See also* gigabyte.

memory   The work area inside your computer that the central processing unit uses to hold data when you run a program.

memory card   A small portable device used to store data.

memory card reader   A device that offers several slots, each of which is designed to hold a particular type of memory card.

menu bar   A horizontal strip that runs across a program window and contains words such as File, Edit, and View (representing the program's pull-down menus).

message body   The text of an email message.

microprocessor   *See* central processing unit.

modem   An electronic device that somehow manages to transmit and receive computer data over telephone lines. Modems come in three flavors: external, internal, and PC Card.

modifier key   A key such as Ctrl, Alt, or Shift that you hold down while you press another key such as a letter, number, or function key to create a key combination.

monitor   The screen on which the computer displays its text, images, and other data.

mouse   A hand-operated pointing device that you use to select things on the screen that you want to work with, as well as to move things here and there on the screen.

mouse pointer   A small arrow that appears on the screen that moves when you move your mouse.

multimedia Digital photos, music, and videos.

multitasking The capability to run two or more programs at the same time.

news portal A website that gathers news stories from a large number of online news sources.

notification A message that pops up in Windows's notification area to let you know when something important is happening with your computer.

operating system The software that controls the overall operation of your computer. Windows is an example of an operating system.

option buttons Dialog box controls that offer mutually exclusive choices so only one option button can be active at a time.

option mark In a pull-down menu, a small dot that appears to the left of the active command in a group of commands, where only one can be active at a time.

page *See* web page.

patch To install any and all Windows updates that Microsoft makes available.

pixels The individual pinpoints of light that make up everything you see on your screen.

phishing A scam that uses bogus email messages and websites to fool you into submitting sensitive or private data, financial information, or a password.

photo-sharing site A website that enables you to share photos with friends and family.

point To move the mouse pointer over a specified part of the screen.

POP (Post Office Protocol)   A set of technologies that enable you to download email messages to your computer.

POP3 server   The mail server that your ISP uses to process email sent to you.

port   A receptacle in the back of a computer into which you plug the cable used by an external device.

portal   A website that aggregates a large collection of related stories and links. *See also* news portal and shopping portal.

printable coupon   A coupon image on a website that you print out and redeem at a real-world store.

processor   *See* central processing unit.

program file   A file that runs an application installed on your computer.

program window   A window that contains a running program.

promotional code   *See* coupon code.

pull-down menu   A list of commands offered by a program.

RAM   *See* memory.

random access memory   *See* memory.

restore point   A snapshot of your computer's current state and configuration.

ribbon   In programs such as Paint, WordPad, and Windows Live Mail, a special type of toolbar that organizes commands into tabs and offers a wider selection of options than a regular toolbar.

right-click   To click the right mouse button instead of the usual left button. In Windows, right-clicking something usually pops up a shortcut menu.

rip To copy tracks from a music CD to your computer.

scale To make text and images appear larger while still preserving text and image clarity.

scanner A photocopier-like device that creates a digital image of a flat surface, such as a piece of paper or a photograph.

screen resolution The number of columns and rows in the grid of pixels that Windows uses to display screen images.

service pack A Windows update that includes problem fixes, security enhancements, new features, and other changes designed to make Windows run better.

shilling In an online auction, using fake bids to drive up the price of an item to an artificially high level.

shopping portal A website that gathers a list of online retailers who sell a particular product.

shortcut menu A menu that contains a few commands related to an item (such as the desktop or the taskbar). You display the shortcut menu by right-clicking the object.

slider A dialog box control that you click and drag to set the value of the setting.

SMTP (Simple Mail Transfer Protocol) A set of technologies that enable you to send email messages from your computer.

SMTP server The mail server that your ISP uses to process email that you send.

social networking An internet service that enables you to share information with family, friends, and people who have similar hobbies and interests.

spam *See* junk email.

spam filter A tool that attempts to separate junk email messages from regular messages and to segregate junk email in a separate folder.

spyware A program that surreptitiously monitors your computer activities or steals sensitive information from your computer.

status bar A horizontal strip along the bottom of a window that a program uses to display information about the current state of the program.

subject line A line of text that describes what an email message is about.

surf To jump from web page to web page using a web browser.

system A computer, as a whole.

system repair disc A special CD or DVD that you can use to recover a computer that will not start.

system unit *See* computer case.

system volume The volume that Windows uses for every audio feature on your computer.

tab In a dialog box, an area of text across the top of the dialog box that displays a new set of controls when clicked; in a web browser, a window within the main browser window that displays a separate web page.

tag A word or short phrase that describes a set of imported photos.

taskbar The gray strip along the bottom of the Windows screen that's used to switch between running programs.

text box A dialog box control in which you enter text.

theme A collection of color schemes that apply all at once to text, windows, the desktop, and other screen elements.

thumb drive *See* flash drive.

thumbnail A scaled-down preview of a photo or other type of file.

title bar The horizontal strip along the top of a window that tells you the name of the program and sometimes the name of the open document.

toolbar A collection of easily accessible icons designed to give you push-button access to common commands and features.

tower case A style of computer case that's tall with a relatively narrow base. *See also* desktop case.

troubleshooter A Windows feature that offers a step-by-step procedure for solving a problem.

tweet A text message sent to Twitter.

uninstall To completely remove a program from your computer.

upload To send data to a remote computer. *See also* download.

upload speed The rate at which your ISP sends data from your computer to the internet, which is usually slower than download speed.

URL The address of a web page.

USB A relatively new way to connect all kinds of devices—including keyboards, mice, speakers, printers, modems, and network cards—to a PC. Most new computers have one or two USB ports into which these devices connect.

virus A software program that installs itself on your computer without you knowing it, then proceeds to steal or destroy data or crash or hijack your computer.

web browser A program that you use to surf sites on the World Wide Web. The browser that comes with Windows is called Internet Explorer.

web page A document on the web that contains text, images, and usually a few links.

website A collection of web pages that appear within a single domain name.

Wi-Fi Short for "wireless fidelity"; a technology that enables you to access the internet without a physical connection to a modem.

wireless router A device that offers wireless internet access by connecting directly to a broadband modem.

Online Resources for Seniors

Appendix B

AARP

www.aarp.org   The online home of the American Association of Retired Persons (AARP; see Figure B.1) offers tons of articles on health, food, travel, money, and much more.

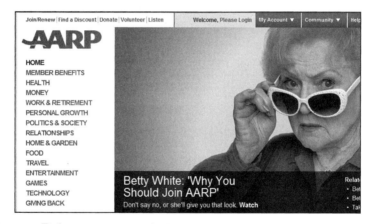

Figure B.1: AARP's website is a great place to start your senior-related surfing safari.

CaregiverList

www.caregiverlist.com   This terrific site offers resources for both seniors and caregivers, including nursing home ratings, senior services by state, and handy checklists for matters such as home care and senior driving.

CaregiverStress

www.caregiverstress.com   This site is aimed mostly at people who provide care for seniors, so it's a great resource if you're caring for a spouse, another senior family member, or a friend.

Grandparents.com

www.grandparents.com   This online magazine (see Figure B.2) is the site to surf for all things grandparental.

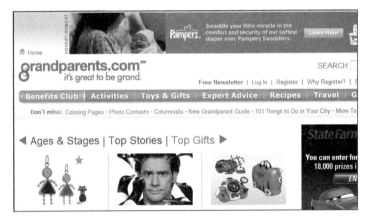

Figure B.2: If you're a grandparent, be sure to check out grandparents.com for lots of useful information.

Healthy Aging

www.cdc.gov/aging/   This great site is maintained by the Centers for Disease Control and Prevention and is loaded with fantastic information on keeping your body and mind healthy as you age.

Merck Manual: Older People's Health Issues

www.merckmanuals.com/home/sec26.html   This page provides tons of great material on senior health, straight from the pages of the famous *Merck Manual.*

NIHSeniorHealth

nihseniorhealth.gov   The National Institutes of Health (NIH) have put together this site, which offers lots of truly useful information on senior health issues.

Retirement Living Information Center

www.retirementliving.com   This useful site offers lots of useful links related to senior living options, including retirement communities, senior-living facilities, state taxes, news, and more.

Senior Citizens' Resources: USA.gov

www.usa.gov/Topics/Seniors.shtml   This U.S. government site (see Figure B.3) offers a wealth of government resources for seniors, including topics related to consumer protection, volunteering, health care, housing, finances, retirement, and travel.

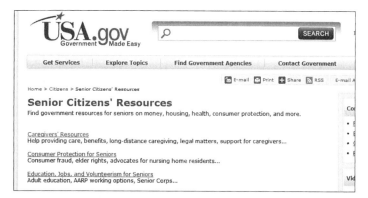

Figure B.3: USA.gov's Senior Citizens' Resources site is bursting with links to useful U.S. government resources.

seniorDECISION

www.seniordecision.com   This site offers ratings and reviews for senior-care facilities and senior housing.

Seniors Canada

www.seniors.gc.ca   This site (see Figure B.4) is maintained by the government of Canada and is home to an impressive collection of links to senior-related information, services, publications, news, and much more.

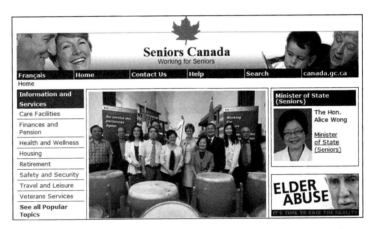

Figure B.4: The Canadian government's Seniors Canada site will keep you busy with a fistful of links to resources.

Seniors Guide Online

www.seniorsguideonline.com   If you're looking for anything from assisted living to financial planning to medical equipment, this useful site can help you locate products and services in your area.

ThirdAge

www.thirdage.com   This fun online magazine celebrates the senior lifestyle with a special focus on women.

Index

Numbers

419 scams, 347-349

A

Acceleration slider, 174
accounts, Facebook, 284-286
Action Center window, 309
Ad-Aware, 308
Add a Favorite dialog box, 226
Add an E-mail Account Wizard, 244
address/search bar (Internet Explorer window), 223
addresses (web), 225
adjustments, volume, 159
    application volume, 161-162
    balancing headphones, 163-164
    Loudness Equalization, 164-165
    system volume, 160
administration passwords, 216
advance fee fraud, 347
Airfare Watchdog, 273
airlines, 273
All Programs icon, 50-51
AllRecipes, 240
Alt key, 34
Amazon, 265
Ancestor Hunt, 238
Ancestry, 238
anti-phishing tools, 341-344
antivirus programs, 230, 300-302
ASDL (Asymmetric Digital Subscriber Line), 202
Asymmetric Digital Subscriber Line (ASDL), 202
attachments, 252-254, 257
auctions, online, 352-354
audio
    connecting sound system, 17-18
    hearing challenges, 157
        speakers/headphones, 158-159
        visual cues for sounds, 165-168
        volume adjustments, 159-165
    Narrator, 154-156
audio CDs, 106-108
automatic arrangement of windows, 177-179
Automatic Backup feature, 116
AutoPlay dialog box, 85
Avast! Antivirus, 300
AVG Internet Security, 300

B

Back button (Internet Explorer window), 223
backing up computer, 114
    configuring backup, 116-117
    creating system repair discs, 118
    external hard drives, 115
Backspace key, 71
Backup and Restore window, 116
backups, 135-137
Balance dialog box, 163
balancing headphones, 163-164
bandwidth, 200
Basic Information section (Facebook), 286
Become, 266
behind-the-ear (BTE) hearing aids, 158
bid shielding, 353
Bing, 231
Bing Maps, 234
Bing News, 237
bitmap file formats, 92
bits, 198
blind courtesy copy, 250
Blocked Senders list, 335-336
blocking pop-ups, 317-319
Bounce Keys feature, 184-185
broadband connections, 197
    equipment, 202-204
    setup, 204-210
browsers, Internet Explorer, 220-223
    downloading files, 229-230
    Favorites feature, 226-228
    navigation, 224-226
    searching for information, 230-231
    tabs, 228-229
browsing history, 313-316
BTE (behind-the-ear) hearing aids, 158
burning photos, 104-105

buttons
    Back, 223
    Close, 65
    Command, 60
    Forward, 223
    New Tab, 228
    Option, 61
    Paint, 74
    Restart, 38
    Shut Down, 37
    Sleep, 37
    Start (taskbar), 31
    Uninstall, 46
    Uninstall/Change, 45
    Voice Settings, 155
buying products (online shopping), 270-271
bytes of data, 10

C

camcorders, 24-25
caption bars, 167
cases (computer), 4-9, 13
CD/DVD disc drives, 21-22
CDs
    audio, 106-108
    copying photos to, 104-105
    disc drives, 21-22
Centers for Disease Control and Prevention, 240
central processing units (CPUs), 9
check boxes, 61
check overpayment scams, 354
CHOW, 240
click (mouse maneuvers), 33
click and drag (mouse maneuvers), 34
ClickLock feature, 174, 176

Close button, 65
closing
    documents, 79
    programs, 64-65, 121
CNET, 265
CNET Shopper, 267
Command button, 60
commands, 55
    Copy, 71
    Cut, 71
    Exit, 65
    New, 68
    Paste, 71
    Refresh, 56
    Save, 74
    Save As, 78
    Sort By, 56
    Status Bar, 56
    Undo, 70, 72
CompactFlash memory card, 23
components
    CD/DVD disc drives, 21-22
    computer cases, 4-9, 13
    connections, 12-13
        keyboards, 16-17
        monitors, 14-15
        mouse, 16-17
        power cords, 20
        printers, 17
        sound systems, 17-18
        USB devices, 19-20
    digital camera connections, 24-25
    external hard drives, 25-26
    flash drives, 24
    hard drives, 10
    keyboards, 5
    media players, 25
    memory, 10
    memory cards, 23
    monitors, 5
    mouse, 5
    processors, 9

composition, email messages, 249-250
computer cases, 4-9, 13
configuration
    backups, 116-117
    Facebook profile, 286-287
    Narrator settings, 155
    wireless routers, 214-217
Connect automatically check box, 210
connections
    computer components, 12-13
        keyboards, 16-17
        monitors, 14-15
        mouse, 16-17
        power cords, 20
        printers, 17
        sound systems, 17-18
        USB devices, 19-20
    digital cameras/camcorders, 24-25
    Internet equipment
        broadband connections, 202-204
        dial-up connections, 201
    media players, 25
    wireless, 211-217
Consumer Reports, 264
Consumer Search, 264
Contacts list (email), 251-252
content area (Internet Explorer window), 223
Control Panel icon, 50
Control Panel window, 144
controls, 60, 98
cookies, 315
Cooking Light, 240
cooking sites, 239-240
Copy command, 71
copying
    highlighted text, 71
    photos, 104-105
Coupon Cabin, 275
Coupon Mom, 275
Coupon Shack, 275

coupons, 274-277
CPUs (central processing units), 9
Craigslist, 268
crashes (programs), 130-132
Create Folder dialog box, 259
creating
　copies of documents, 78
　documents, 68-69
　folders, 77-78
　system repair discs, 118
credit card security, 312-313
credit reports, 346
cropping photos, 103-104
Ctrl key, 34
Current Codes, 275
Cut command, 71

D

data bytes, 10
date and time (taskbar), 31
default folders (Windows Live Mail), 248-249
Default Programs icon, 50
Delete Browsing History dialog box, 314
Delete key, 71
Deleted Items default folder (Windows Live Mail), 249
deleting
　browsing history, 313-316
　email messages, 257-259
　text, 71
desktop
　computer cases, 13
　Windows screen, 30
Device and System Sounds volume controls, 162
Devices and Printers icon, 50

DHCP Internet connection, 216
dial-up connections, 197-199
　equipment, 201
　setup, 204-210
dialog boxes, 57-62
　Add a Favorite, 226
　AutoPlay, 85
　Balance, 163
　Create Folder, 259
　Delete Browsing History, 314
　Download Complete, 229
　File Download—Security Warning, 41
　Import Photos and Videos, 86-87, 91
　Internet Options, 222
　Microsoft SmartScreen Filter, 343
　Open, 253
　Safety Options, 330
　Select a System Image Backup, 137
　Sound, 163
　System Recovery Options, 137
　User Account Control, 307
　visual challenges, 152-153
digital cameras, 84
　connections, 24-25
　transferring photos to computer, 84-88
directions, mapping sites, 234-235
discs, system repair, 118
documents, 49
　closing, 79
　creating, 68-69
　defined, 68
　editing, 69-72
　enlarging text, 142
　　Magnifier, 147-148
　　scaling screen, 144-147
　　screen resolution, 142-144
　locating, 80-81
　opening, 79-80

saving, 73
    creating copies of documents, 78
    creating folders, 77-78
    existing documents, 75
    new documents, 74-75
    organization of documents, 76-77
Documents icon, 49
domain names, 225
double-click (mouse maneuvers), 33
Download Complete dialog box, 229
download speed, 200
downloading files, 229-230
Drafts default folder (Windows Live Mail), 248
dragging mouse (ClickLock feature), 174-176
drives
    CD/DVD, 6
    CD/DVD discs, 21-22
    external hard drives, 25-26, 115
    flash, 24
drop-down list boxes, 61
DVDs
    copying photos to, 104-105
    watching movies, 109-110

E

Ease of Access center, 147
eBay, 268
Edit My Profile link (Facebook), 286
editing
    documents, 69-72
    photos, 99
        cropping, 103-104
        removal of red eye, 101-102
        straightening, 100
Edmunds, 265

email
    phishing scams, 339-342
    security, 321
        Blocked Senders, 335-336
        hoaxes, 332-334
        Safe Senders, 334-335
        spam, 325-332
        viruses, 322-325
    Windows Live Mail
        account setup, 244-247
        default folders, 248-249
        receiving email, 254-260
        sending email, 249-254
engines (search), 230
enlarging mouse pointer, 151
enlarging text, 142
    Magnifier, 147-148
    scaling screen, 144-147
    screen resolution, 142-144
Epicurious, 240
Epinions, 265
equalization of volume, 164-165
Equifax, 346
equipment
    CD/DVD disc drives, 21-22
    computer cases, 4-9, 13
    connections, 12-13
        keyboards, 16-17
        monitors, 14-15
        mouse, 16-17
        power cords, 20
        printers, 17
        sound systems, 17-18
        USB devices, 19-20
    digital camera connections, 24-25
    external hard drives, 25-26
    flash drives, 24
    hard drives, 10

Internet connections
  broadband connections, 202-204
  dial-up connections, 201
keyboards, 5
media players, 25
memory, 10
memory cards, 23
monitors, 5
mouse, 5
processors, 9
ergonomics, 12
error messages, 119
Esc key, 35
existing documents
  opening, 79-80
  saving, 75
Exit command, 65
Expedia, 271
Experian, 346
extended keyboards, 35
external hard drives, 25-26, 115

F

Facebook, 282
  setup, 283
    account creation, 284-286
    friends, 287-293
    profile configuration, 286-287
    status updates, 293-294
  sharing links, 295-296
  sharing photos, 295
FamilyLink, 238
FamilySearch, 238
Favorites feature, 226-228
File Download—Security Warning dialog box, 41

file formats, 92-94
files
  downloading, 229-230
  email attachments, 253-254
  recovery, 128-130
Filter Keys feature, 183-184
filters (spam), 329-332
Find a Grave, 238
Find and fix problems link, 122
Firewall (Windows), 303-304
flash drives, 24
Flickr, 233
Flight Center, 271
folders, 49
  creating, 77-78
  default, 248-249
  storing email messages, 259-260
Food Network, 240
Food & Wine, 240
Forward button (Internet Explorer window), 223
forwarding email messages, 257-259
fraud, online shopping, 349
  auctions, 352-354
  bogus health products, 354-355
  check overpayment scams, 354
  free offers, 355-356
  payment options, 350-352
fridge Googling, 239-240
friends
  Facebook, 287-293
  social networking, 279-280
    Facebook, 283-296
    selection, 281-283
front access ports, 7

G

Genealogy, 238
genealogy sites, 238
general fixes, troubleshooting problems, 121-123
Geni, 238
GIF file formats, 92
gigabytes, 10
Good Housekeeping, 265
Google, 231
Google+, 282
Google Maps, 234
Google News, 237
Google Product Search, 267
graphics programs, 59
Grocery Coupon Network, 275
group coupons, 276
Groupon, 277

H

hard disks, 10
hard drives
    capacities, 10
    external, 25-26, 115
hardware
    CD/DVD disc drives, 21-22
    computer cases, 4-9, 13
    connections, 12-13
        keyboards, 16-17
        monitor, 14-15
        mouse, 16-17
        power cords, 20
        printer, 17
        sound system, 17-18
        USB devices, 19-20
    digital camera connections, 24-25
    external hard drives, 25-26
    flash drives, 24
    hard drives, 10
    keyboards, 5
    media players, 25
    memory, 10
    memory cards, 23
    monitors, 5
    mouse, 5
    processors, 9
headphones
    balancing, 163-164
    hearing challenges, 158-159
health information, 240-241
health products, 354-355
hearing challenges, 157
    speakers/headphones, 158-159
    visual cues for sounds, 165
        Sound Sentry, 166-167
        text captions for spoken dialog, 167-168
    volume adjustments, 159
        application volume, 161-162
        balancing headphones, 163-164
        Loudness Equalization, 164-165
        system volume, 160
Help and Support icon, 50
My Heritage, 238
high-contrast screens, 149-150
high-contrast themes, 149
highlighting text, 70
HTTP servers, 245

I

iChef, 240
icons, 47
    programs (taskbar), 31
    Start menu, 49-50

identity theft, 345-347
IMAP servers, 245
Import Pictures and Videos dialog box, 86-87, 91
in-the-ear (ITE) hearing aids, 158
Inbox default folder (Windows Live Mail), 248
information searching, 230-231
InPrivate browsing, 316-317
input devices
    keyboards, 34-36
    mouse, 31-34
installation of programs, 40-43
Installed Updates window, 120
Internet Explorer
    anti-phishing tools, 343-344
    connections
        broadband connections, 202-204
        dial-up connections, 201
        setup, 204-210
        wireless connections, 211-217
    disconnecting, 211
    downloading files, 229-230
    Favorites feature, 226-228
    genealogy sites, 238
    health information, 240-241
    Internet Explorer, 220-223
        downloading files, 229-230
        Favorites feature, 226-228
        navigation, 224-226
        searching for information, 230-231
        tabs, 228-229
    mapping sites, 234-235
    navigation, 224-226
    online news, 235-237
    online shopping, 261-262
        coupons, 274-277
        research, 263-270
        transactions, 270-271
        trip-planning resources, 271-274

    recipe sites, 239-240
    searching for information, 230-231
    security, 299
        blocking pop-ups, 317-319
        credit cards, 312-313
        deletion of browsing history, 313-316
        email, 321-336
        general surfing tips, 307-309
        InPrivate browsing, 316-317
        passwords, 310-312
        scams, 337-356
        spyware, 303-305
        UAC (User Account Control), 306-307
        viruses, 300-302
    service providers, 196-197
        broadband connections, 200
        dial-up connections, 198-199
    sharing photos, 232-234
    tabs, 228-229
    wireless connections, 211-217
Internet Options dialog box, 222
ISPs (Internet service providers), 196-197
    broadband connections, 200
    dial-up connections, 198-199
ITE (in-the-ear) hearing aids, 158

J

JPEG file formats, 93
jump lists, 48
junk email, 325-328
Junk Email default folder (Windows Live Mail), 248
junk emailers, 326

K

key combinations, 34
keyboards, 5
    connections, 16-17
    highlighting text, 70
    maneuvers, 34-36
    moving mouse, 170-174
    physical challenges, 179
        Bounce Keys feature, 184-185
        Filter Keys feature, 183-184
        Repeat Keys feature, 185-186
        Slow Keys feature, 185-186
        Sticky Keys feature, 180-182
        unwanted keystrokes, 183
    ports, 8
    shortcuts, 148, 180-182
    wireless, 16
keystrokes
    multiple
        Bounce Keys feature, 184-185
        Repeat Keys feature, 185-186
        Slow Keys feature, 185-186
    unwanted, 183-184
kilobytes, 10

L

launching programs, 46-53
libraries, 76
line jack (modems), 201
LinkedIn, 282
links
    Find and fix problems, 122
    sharing on Facebook, 295-296
    web pages, 220-224
List Box control, 62

Live Mail (Windows)
    account setup, 244-247
    anti-phishing tools, 341-342
    antivirus settings, 323-325
    default folders, 248-249
    receiving email, 254
        attachments, 257
        reading messages, 255-256
        replies/forwards, 257-259
        storing messages, 259-260
    sending email, 249
        attachments, 252-254
        composition, 249-250
        Contacts list, 251-252
LivingSocial, 277
locating documents, 80-81
logging off Windows, 121
loss leader, 349
lost files, 128-130
Loudness Equalization, 164-165
Loudness Equalization check box, 165

M

magazine sites, 237
Magnifier, 147-148
mail servers, 245
Make the Mouse Easier to Use window, 174
MapQuest, 234
maps, 234-235
McAfee antivirus program, 230
McAfee Internet Security Suite, 300
media players, 25
megabytes, 10
memory, 10
memory cards, 23, 84
    readers, 6
    transferring photos to computer, 90-91

menu bars, 54
menus
    pull-down, 53-57
    shortcut, 33
    Start, 46-50
    View, 54
message body (email), 250
microprocessors, 9
Microsoft Knowledge Base, 124
Microsoft Password Checker, 311
Microsoft Product Support Services, 124
Microsoft SmartScreen Filter dialog box, 343
MMC (MultiMedia Card), 23
modems
    broadband, 202
    line jacks, 201
    ports, 8
    telephone jacks, 201
modifier keys, 180
monitors, 5
    connections, 14-15
    ports, 8
mouse, 5
    connections, 16-17
    enlarging pointer, 151
    highlighting text, 70
    maneuvers, 31-34
    physical challenges, 170
        ClickLock feature, 174-176
        Mouse Keys feature, 170-174
        prevention of window arrangement, 177-179
        window selection, 176-177
    pointer, 32
    ports, 8
Mouse Keys feature, 170-174
Mouse pointers box, 151
movies, 109-110
moving
    email messages, 257-259
    highlighted text, 71
    mouse
        ClickLock feature, 174-176
        Mouse Keys feature, 170-174
        prevention of window arrangement, 177-179
        window selection, 176-177
MSN.com website, 221
MultiMedia Card (MMC), 23
multiple keystrokes
    Bounce Keys feature, 184-185
    Repeat Keys feature, 185-186
    Slow Keys feature, 185-186
music
    audio CDs, 106-107
    copying music from audio CDs, 107-108
Music icon, 49
MySpace, 283

N

Narrator, 154-156
National Institutes of Health, 240
navigation
    Start menu, 50-53
    web pages, 224-226
Network and Sharing Center window, 206
Network Map window, 215
networks
    cables, 203
    ports, 8
New command, 68
New Connection Wizard, 208
new documents, 74-75
New Message window, 249

New Tab button, 228
news portals, 237
news sites, 235-237
NewsIsFree, 237
niche networks, 281
Nigerian letter scams, 347-349
noise-canceling headphones, 159
Norton antivirus program, 230
Norton Internet Security, 300
"Not Responding" text, 130
notification area (taskbar), 31
notifications, 186-188
Num Lock feature, 35, 171
numeric keypads, 35, 172

O

offensive messages, 326
online services
    connecting Internet equipment, 201
        broadband connections, 202-204
        dial-up connections, 201
    disconnecting Internet, 211
    genealogy sites, 238
    health information, 240-241
    Internet Explorer, 220-223
        downloading files, 229-230
        Favorites feature, 226-228
        navigation, 224-226
        searching for information, 230-231
        tabs, 228-229
    Internet service providers, 196-197
        broadband connections, 200
        dial-up connections, 198-199
    mapping sites, 234-235
    news sites, 235-237
    recipe sites, 239-240
    security, 299
        blocking pop-ups, 317-319
        credit cards, 312-313
        deletion of browsing history, 313-316
        email, 321-336
        general surfing tips, 307-309
        InPrivate browsing, 316-317
        passwords, 310-312
        scams, 337-356
        spyware, 303-305
        UAC (User Account Control), 306-307
        viruses, 300-302
    sharing photos, 232-234
    shopping, 261-262
        coupons, 274-277
        fraud, 349-356
        research, 263-270
        transactions, 270-271
        trip-planning resources, 271-274
    troubleshooting resources, 124-125
    wireless connections to Internet, 211-217
Open dialog box, 253
opening documents, 79-80
operating systems, Windows
    input devices, 31
        keyboard, 34-36
        mouse, 31-34
    logging off, 121
    screens, 29-31
    troubleshooters, 122-123
Option button, 61
option marks, 56
Orbitz, 272
organization
    saving documents, 76-77
    work area, 11-12
Orkut, 281
Outbox default folder (Windows Live Mail), 249

P

page title (Internet Explorer window), 223
pages (web), 219
    downloading files, 229-230
    Favorites feature, 226-228
    links, 220-224
    navigation, 224-226
    searching for information, 230-231
    tabs, 228-229
Paint, 59
Paint button, 74
parts of computer
    CD/DVD disc drives, 21-22
    computer cases, 4-9, 13
    connections, 12-13
        keyboards, 16-17
        monitors, 14-15
        mouse, 16-17
        power cords, 20
        printers, 17
        sound systems, 17-18
        USB devices, 19-20
    digital camera connections, 24-25
    external hard drives, 25-26
    flash drives, 24
    hard drives, 10
    keyboards, 5
    media players, 25
    memory, 10
    memory cards, 23
    monitors, 5
    mouse, 5
    processors, 9
Password Checker (Microsoft), 311
passwords, 21, 216, 310-312
Paste command, 71
pasting highlighted text, 71
patching PCs, 308

payment options, online shopping, 350-352
PayPal, 351
Personalization window, 149
phishing, 327, 338
    anti-phishing tools, 343-344
    email messages, 339-342
    websites, 342-344
Photobucket, 233
photos
    burning to CD/DVD, 104-105
    editing, 99
        cropping, 103-104
        removal of red eye, 101-102
        straightening, 100
    email attachments, 252-253
    file formats, 92-94
    sharing, 232-234, 295
    transferring to computer
        digital cameras, 84-88
        memory cards, 90-91
        scanners, 88-89
    viewing, 94
        previews, 95-97
        slide shows, 98-99
physical challenges, 169
    keyboards 179
        Bounce Keys feature, 184-185
        Filter Keys feature, 183-184
        Repeat Keys feature, 185-186
        Slow Keys feature, 185-186
        Sticky Keys feature, 180-182
        unwanted keystrokes, 183
    mouse, 170
        ClickLock feature, 174-176
        Mouse Keys feature, 170-174
        prevention of window arrangement, 177-179
        window selection, 176-177
    notifications, 186-188
    voice commands, 188-191

Picasa Web Albums, 233
Pictures icon, 49
Pictures library, 95
Pin the Favorites Center icon, 228
pixels, 142
PNG file formats, 93
point (mouse maneuvers), 32
Pop-up Blocker, 318
pop-up windows, 317-319
POP3 servers, 245
portals, 221, 266
ports
    front access, 7
    keyboards, 8
    modems, 8
    monitors, 8
    mouse, 8
    networks, 8
    sound, 8
    USB, 8
power cords, 20
power outlets, 8
power switches, 7
PPPoE Internet connection, 216
PriceGrabber, 267
Priceline, 273
Print Screen key, 271
printable coupons, 275
printers, 17
processors, 9
product pitches, 326
products, online shopping, 263-265
profiles (Facebook), 286-287
Program Compatibility troubleshooter, 122
programs
    antivirus, 230, 300-302
    closing, 64-65, 121
    dialog boxes, 60-62
    icons (taskbar), 31
    installation, 40-43
    launching, 46-53
    Paint, 59
    pull-down menus, 53-57
    recovery from crashes, 130-132
    switching between, 62-64
    toolbars, 57
    uninstalling, 44-46
    WordPad, 59
promotional codes, 274-275
protection level, spam filters, 329-332
Public Health Agency of Canada, 240
pull-down menus, 53-57

Q-R

Quick Views default folder (Windows Live Mail), 248

RAM (random access memory), 10
Rand McNally, 234
random access memory (RAM), 10
Ravelry, 281
RCA-style jack, 17
readers, memory cards, 6
reading email messages, 255-256
receiving email, 254-255
    attachments, 257
    reading messages, 255-256
    replies/forwards, 257-259
    storing messages, 259-260
recipe sites, 239-240
recovery (troubleshooting problems), 128
    backups, 135-137
    lost files, 128-130
    program crashes, 130-132
    System Restore, 133-135
Red eye tool (photo editing), 101-102
Refresh command, 56
Remote Assistance (Windows), 126-128
remote control, 125-128

removal of red eye (photos), 101-102
repair discs, 118
Repeat Keys feature, 185-186
replying to email messages, 257-259
Requires authentication check box, 247
research, online shopping, 263
    prices, 266-268
    products, 263-265
    retailers, 268-270
ResellerRatings, 269
resources
    health information, 240-241
    troubleshooting problems
        online resources, 124-125
        remote control route, 125-128
Restart button, 38
restarting computer, 38, 121
Restore Files wizard, 129
restore points, 133
retailers, online shopping research, 268-270
RetailMeNot, 275
ribbon, 59
right-click (mouse maneuvers), 33
ripping CD tracks, 107
RootsWeb, 238
routers, wireless, 212-217

S

Safe Mode, 133
Safe Senders list (email security), 334-335
safety. *See* security
Safety Options dialog box, 330
Save As command, 78
Save command, 74
saving documents, 73
    creating copies, 78
    creating folders, 77-78
    existing documents, 75
    new documents, 74-75
    organization of documents, 76-77

scaling screen, 144-147
Scam Busters, 333
scams, 337
    419, 347-349
    identity theft, 345-347
    junk email, 327
    online shopping fraud, 349
        auctions, 352-354
        bogus health products, 354-355
        check overpayment scams, 354
        free offers, 355-356
        payment options, 350-352
    phishing, 338
        email messages, 339-342
        websites, 342-344
    Scam Busters, 333
Scanner and Camera Wizard, 88
scanners, 84, 88-89
screens, 5
    high-contrast, 149-150
    resolution, 142-144
    scaling, 144-147
    zooming in, 147-148
    Windows, 29-31
scripts, 323
scroll (mouse maneuvers), 34
search engines, 230-231
Search text box (Facebook), 288
SeatGuru, 274
security
    backing up computer, 114
        configuring backup, 116-117
        creating system repair discs, 118
        external hard drives, 115
    blocking pop-ups, 317-319
    credit cards, 312-313
    deletion of browsing history, 313-316
    email, 321
        Blocked Senders, 335-336
        hoaxes, 332-334
        Safe Senders, 334-335
        spam, 325-332
        viruses, 322-325

Index

general surfing tips, 307-309
InPrivate browsing, 316-317
passwords, 310-312
scams, 337
    419, 347-349
    identity theft, 345-347
    online shopping fraud, 349-356
    phishing, 338-344
spyware, 303-305
UAC (User Account Control), 306-307
viruses, 300-302
wireless networks, 216
Security Check page (Facebook), 285
Select a System Image Backup dialog box, 137
sending email
    attachments, 252-254
    composition, 249-250
    Contacts list, 251-252
Sent Items default folder (Windows Live Mail), 248
service packs, 121
service providers (Internet), 196-197
    broadband connections, 200
    dial-up connections, 198-199
Set up Speech Recognition Wizard, 189
Set Up Windows Internet Explorer 8 Wizard, 221
setup
    CD/DVD disc drives, 21-22
    component connections, 12-13
        keyboards, 16-17
        monitors, 14-15
        mouse, 16-17
        power cords, 20
        printers, 17
        sound system, 17-18
        USB devices, 19-20
    computer cases, 4-9
    digital camera connections, 24-25
    external hard drives, 25-26
    Facebook, 283
        account creation, 284-286
        friends, 287-293

        profile configuration, 286-287
        sharing links, 295-296
        sharing photos, 295
        status updates, 293-294
    flash drives, 24
    hard drives, 10
    Internet connections, 204-210
    keyboards, 5
    media players, 25
    memory, 10
    memory cards, 23
    monitors, 5
    mouse, 5
    organization of work area, 11-12
    processors, 9
    Windows Live Mail, 244-247
    wireless connections, 212-217
sharing
    links (Facebook), 295-296
    photos, 232-234, 295
Shift key, 34
shill bidding, 353
shopping online
    fraud, 349
        auctions, 352-354
        bogus health products, 354-355
        check overpayment scams, 354
        free offers, 355-356
        payment options, 350-352
    portals, 266
Shopzilla, 268
shortcut menus, 33
shortcuts, keyboard
    Magnifier, 148
    Sticky Keys feature, 180-182
Show numbers (Speech Recognition), 188
Shut Down button, 37
Shutterfly, 233
shutting down computer, 36-37
Sign Up section (Facebook), 284
Simply Recipes, 240
Sleep button, 37

slide shows, 98-99
Slider control, 62
Slow Keys feature, 185-186
SmartScreen Filter, 343
SMTP servers, 245
Snapfish, 233
Snopes, 333
social networking, 279
    Facebook, 284
        setup, 283-294
        sharing links, 295-296
        sharing photos, 295
    selection, 281-283
Sort By command, 56
sound
    ports, 8
    visual cues for, 165
        Sound Sentry, 166-167
        text captions for spoken dialog, 167-168
Sound dialog box, 163
Sound Sentry, 166-167
sound systems, 17-18
spam
    email security, 325-328
    filters, 329-332
spammers, 326
speakers
    connections, 17
    hearing challenges, 158-159
Speech Recognition feature, 188-191
Speech Reference Card, 190
speed
    Internet connections, 198
    Mouse Keys feature, 173-174
spoken dialog, text captions, 167-168
Spybot Search & Destroy, 308
spyware, 303
    junk email messages, 327
    Windows Defender, 304-305

Spyware Doctor, 308
Start button (taskbar), 31
Start menu, 46-48
    icons, 49-50
    navigation, 50-53
Start Narrator Minimized check box, 156
starting computer, 20-21
Status Bar command, 56
Status column (Task Manager), 132
status updates (Facebook), 293-294
Sticky Keys feature, 180-182
storing email messages, 259-260
Straighten tool (photo editing), 100-101
submenus, 51
suffixes (domain names), 225
Suspicious Website message, 344
switching between programs, 62-64
system
    images, 135
    repair discs, 118
    unit, 5
    volume, 160
System Protection, 133
System Recovery Options dialog box, 137
System Restore, 133-135

T

Tab control, 62
tabs, 228-229
tags, 86
Task column (Task Manager), 132
Task Manager (Windows), 131-132
taskbars, 30-31, 58
technical support (Microsoft Product Support Services), 124
telecoil mode (hearing aids), 159
telephone jacks (modems), 201

text
  deleting, 71
  enlarging, 142
    Magnifier, 147-148
    scaling screen, 144-147
    screen resolution, 142-144
  highlighting, 70
  "Not Responding," 130
text boxes, 50-61
text captions, 167-168
themes, 149
three-fingered salute, 131
thumb drives, 24
thumbnails, 95
TIF file formats, 93
title bars, 167
toolbars, 57
Tools and Settings window, 305
Top Ten Reviews, 265
tower computer cases, 13
transactions, online shopping, 270-271
transceiver, 16
transferring photos to computer, 84
  digital cameras, 84-88
  memory cards, 90-91
  scanners, 88-89
TransUnion, 346
travel, online trip-planning resources, 271-274
Travelocity, 272
trip-planning resources, 271-274
TripAdvisor, 272
troubleshooting, 119
  backing up computer, 114
    configuring backup, 116-117
    creating system repair discs, 118
    external hard drives, 115
  determining source of problem, 119-121
  general fixes, 121-122

recovery from problems, 128
  backups, 135-137
  lost files, 128-130
  program crashes, 130-132
  System Restore, 133-135
resources, 124
  online resources, 124-125
  remote control route, 125-128
  Windows troubleshooters, 122-123
Turn on ClickLock check box, 175
Turn on Filter Keys check box, 183
Turn on Mouse Keys check box, 171
Turn on Narrator check box, 156
Turn On Pop-up Blocker check box, 318
TV news sites, 236
Twitter, 282

U

U.S. Department of Health and Human Services, 240
UAC (User Account Control), 306-307
Undo command, 70-72
Uniform Resource Locators (URLs), 225
Uninstall button, 46
Uninstall/Change button, 45
uninstalling programs, 44-46
Universal Serial Bus (USB)
  cables, 203
  devices, 19-20
  ports, 8
unwanted keystrokes, 183-184
upload speed, 200
Urban Legends, 333
URLs (Uniform Resource Locators), 225
USB (Universal Serial Bus)
  cables, 203
  devices, 19-20
  ports, 8

Use FilterKeys check box, 184
Use MouseKeys check box, 172
User Account Control dialog box, 307
User Account Control (UAC), 306-307
User name icon, 49

V

vendor websites, 125
Veterans Health Administration, 240
VGA connectors, 14
video display, 5
View menu, 54
viewing photos, 94
   previews, 95-97
   slide shows, 98-99
viruses, 300-302, 322-325
visual challenges, 141
   dialog boxes, 152-153
   enlarging mouse pointer, 151
   enlarging text, 142
      Magnifier, 147-148
      scaling screen, 144-147
      screen resolution, 142-144
   high-contrast screen, 149-150
   Narrator, 154-156
   removal of distractions, 153-154
visual cues for sounds, 165
   Sound Sentry, 166-167
   text captions for spoken dialog, 167-168
voice commands, 189-191
Voice Settings button, 155
volume adjustments, 159
   application volume, 161-162
   balancing headphones, 163-164
   Loudness Equalization, 164-165
   system volume, 160

Volume Mixer, 161
Vulcan nerve pinch, 131

W-X-Y-Z

Web addresses, 225
web browsers (Internet Explorer), 220-223
   downloading files, 229-230
   Favorites feature, 226-228
   navigation, 224-226
   searching for information, 230-231
   tabs, 228-229
web pages, 219
   downloading files, 229-230
   Favorites feature, 226-228
   links, 220-224
   navigation, 224-226
   searching for information, 230-231
   tabs, 228-229
web sites
   phishing scams, 342-344
   photo sharing, 232
web (World Wide Web). *See* Internet Explorer
Webshots, 233
Wi-Fi, 211-213
   router configuration, 214-217
   tapping into connection, 217
windows
   Action Center, 309
   automatic arrangement, 177-179
   Backup and Restore, 116
   Control Panel, 144
   Installed Updates, 120
   Internet Explorer, 222
   Make the Mouse Easier to Use, 174
   Network and Sharing Center, 206

Network Map, 215
New Message, 249
Personalization, 149
pop-ups, 319
selection, 176-177
Tools and Settings, 305
Windows Media Player, 108
Windows (operating system), 27-28
   input devices, 31
      keyboard, 34-36
      mouse, 31-34
   logging off, 121
   screens, 29-31
   troubleshooters, 122-123
Windows Defender, 304-305
Windows Firewall, 303-304
Windows Live Essentials program
   installation, 40-42
   uninstalling, 44-45
Windows Live Mail
   account setup, 244-247
   anti-phishing tools, 341-342
   antivirus settings, 323-325
   default folders, 248-249
   receiving email, 254
      attachments, 257
      reading messages, 255-256
      replies/forwards, 257-259
      storing messages, 259-260
   sending email, 249
      attachments, 252-254
      composition, 249-250
      Contacts list, 251-252
Windows Media Player window, 108
Windows Remote Assistance, 126-128
Windows Task Manager, 131-132
wire-transfer scams, 354

wireless connections, 211-213
   router configuration, 214-217
   tapping into connection, 217
wireless keyboards, 16
wireless routers, 212
wizards
   Add an E-mail Account, 244
   New Connection, 208
   Restore Files, 129
   Scanner and Camera, 88
   Set up Speech Recognition, 189
   Set Up Windows Internet Explorer 8, 221
word processors, 59
WordPad, 59
work space, 11-12
World Wide Web (WWW). *See* Internet Explorer
WWW (World Wide Web). *See* Internet Explorer

Yahoo! Shopping, 268

zooming in on screen, 147-148

CHECK OUT THESE BEST-SELLERS

More than 450 titles available at booksellers and online retailers everywhere!

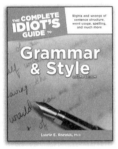
978-1-59257-115-4

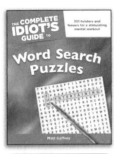
978-1-59257-900-6

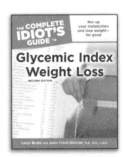
978-1-59257-855-9

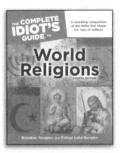
978-1-61564-069-0

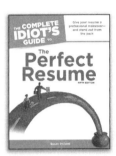
978-1-59257-957-0

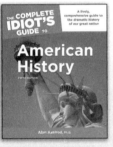
978-1-59257-869-6

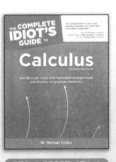
978-1-59257-471-1

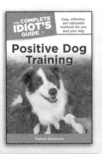
978-1-61564-066-9

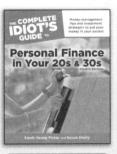
978-1-59257-883-2

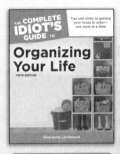
978-1-59257-966-2

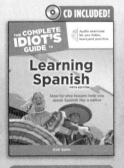
978-1-59257-908-2

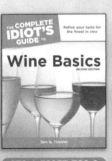
978-1-59257-786-6

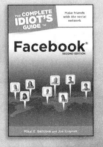
978-1-61564-118-5

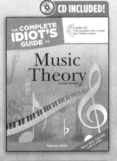
978-1-59257-437-7

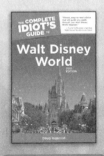
978-1-61564-112-3

 idiotsguides.com